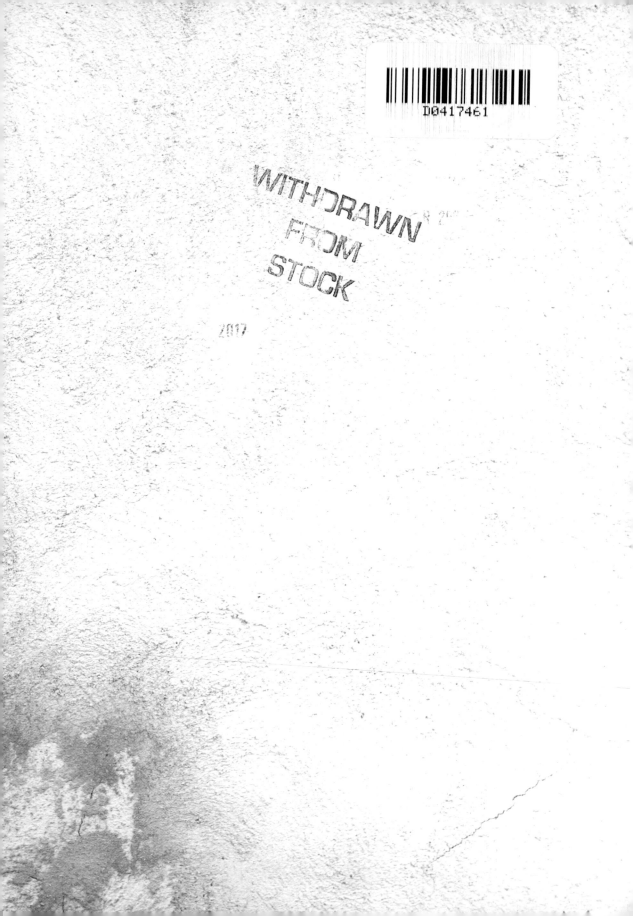

My Life Goals Journal

My Life Goals Journal

Wellness strategies to transform your life

ANDREA HAYES

GILL BOOKS

Gill Books
Hume Avenue
Park West
Dublin 12
www.gillbooks.ie

Gill Books is an imprint of M.H. Gill & Co.

© Andrea Hayes 2016

978 07171 7436 2

Designed by Tanya M Ross, www.elementinc.ie
Printed by B Z Graf, Poland

This book is typeset in Freight 10pt.

The paper used in this book comes from the wood pulp of managed forests. For every tree felled, at least one tree is planted, thereby renewing natural resources.

A CIP catalogue record for this book is available from the British Library.
All photos © iStock.

5 4 3 2 1

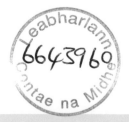

To Brooke

Acknowledgements

I would like to say a big thank you to the team at Gill, and to Sarah Liddy, Vanessa O'Loughlin, Claudia Carroll, Brendan Courtney, Jenny McCarthy and Aidan Storey.

Finally, I would like to thank the readers. I wish them blessings and abundance on their personal life goals journey.

A MESSAGE FROM ANDREA

My Health Journey

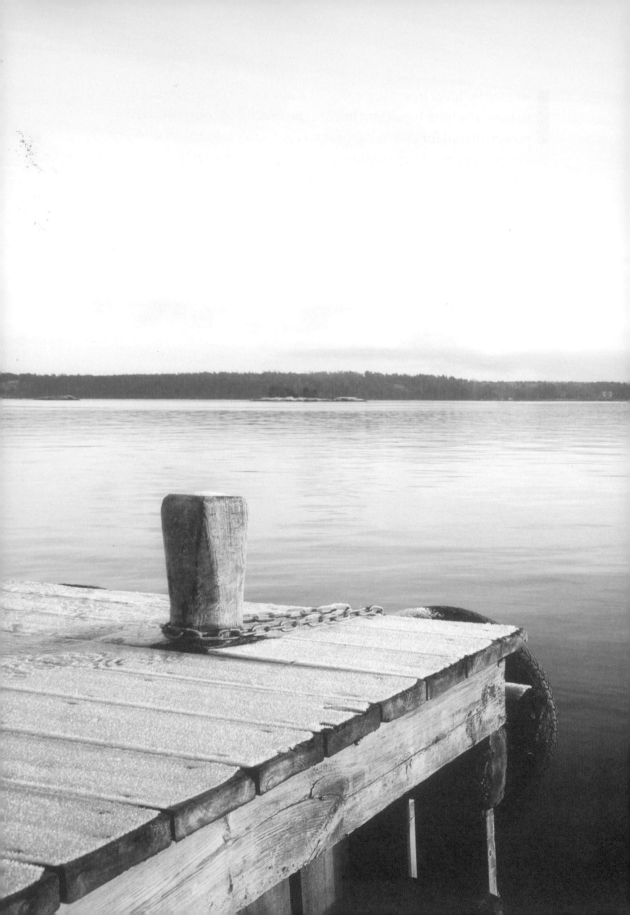

I'm a big believer in setting goals. The first step in goal-setting is to have absolute belief and faith in the process. A journal can be a powerful tool for achieving your goals. The simple practice of writing forces you to reflect on your life, and writing down your thoughts can be a cathartic process. I have created a system that works for me and I know it will work for you, too.

Central to my success is a belief in my ability to absolutely **transform my life**. Making changes in life is not about one-off actions, it is about forming new habits to transform your life. If you follow the month-by-month strategies, I know you can achieve great change. If you want to succeed in any area of your life – personal, professional or even your health – you need to set goals, because without goals you can lack focus.

For me it all started when I made it my intention and goal to live pain free.

Some of you may have read snippets of my story in the press and perhaps have picked up a copy of my memoir, *Pain-Free Life*, and will probably know that I have had 'back pain'. To say it was just back pain minimises it and diminishes the far reach of a complex pain problem that I was desperately trying to manage and, in many ways, keep secret while maintaining a sometimes gruelling TV and media career.

My pain started when I was very young. I have always been, according to my big brother, a sickly sister and have spent various periods of time in hospital since childhood with ear, nose and throat problems. But my ENT issues didn't really hold me back growing up, and I didn't feel any different from anyone else. However, unlike most other people, I have lived with pain in my upper body for most of my life.

My pain story continued into my teens and became much worse after another long hospital stay. I had suspected meningitis and, after a lumbar puncture, I remember feeling the start of what was to become persistent lower back and coccyx pain. But I was a growing teenager and this was passed off as women's problems.

In my twenties I searched for answers for my mysterious pain. I wanted a diagnosis, I wanted a cure – in truth, I wanted help, support and answers. I just wanted to be believed that my pain was real.

Over the years, I took a concoction of medications to manage the pain, threw a potpourri of alternative solutions into the mix and underwent medical procedures but, sadly, the pain persisted – often not as strongly but it was always there.

The anguish and sheer suffering that living in pain causes a person is devastating, and it tore away at the very fabric of my life. On a personal level I felt like a failure. Why couldn't I fix this problem – was I the problem? It was a constant torture that I endured, mentally and physically, daily.

Then one day everything changed. Sometimes we need a push, a nudge from the universe to trust our own inner wisdom to make things happen.

For me, a simple phone call was the catalyst to propel me to follow my own journey to wellness and healing. After spending more than half of my life looking for answers and a name for the constant pain that I have felt since my teens, suddenly, in one moment, had a simple phone call given me an explanation?

It was a Monday morning in December 2013. I was sitting at my desk in TV3, feeling the pressure of a hectic schedule. I was mid-shoot for a one-hour festive TV special called *Coming Home for Christmas* – the whole show had to be filmed, edited and delivered to air on Christmas Eve. Coupled with that I was busy with my weekly radio show on Sunshine 106.8 and voice-over work, and, as it was December, I had also volunteered to cover a few afternoon shifts on a charity radio station called Christmas FM. I was snowed under.

A number flashed up on my mobile and I recognised it immediately as St Vincent's Hospital. Much to my surprise it was my doctor.

I have been attending Dr Paul Murphy for many years for ongoing pain-management procedures but I had never received a call from him, so in hindsight I should probably have listened more carefully or maybe even asked a few questions, but I really couldn't take in quite what he was saying at the time. He told me a rare brain disorder had shown up on my recent MRI scan, and, as if that wasn't troubling enough, the MRI showed more cervical disc degeneration – we would need to discuss it when I saw him that Friday. Perhaps it was shock that made my responses monosyllabic, but, apart from 'Yes, I'll see you Friday', I didn't say anything – I did manage to scrawl 'Chiari malformation 1' on the pad in front of me, though.

The phone call was brief but the impact was huge, not because of the diagnosis but because of what I did next. Instinct kicked in and, although I didn't know anything about the condition Dr Murphy had just outlined, I knew I needed to make a change. So I did something unplanned and very out of character – I asked my line manager in TV3 if I could apply for three months' leave.

And the chain reaction began.

I received an email confirming I could take leave starting in January 2014. Knowing I would have this time off seemed to get me through December. During those weeks I ignored my new diagnosis and what it would mean for my life and my family. But something seismic had shifted inside: I realised I felt numb to everything going on around me; I was just going through the motions, feeling totally out of balance. In truth, I was at breaking point. Taking pill after pill to mask my pain, I desperately struggled through work only to crash and burn at the end of every week. I had no quality of life. I was hopelessly trying to stay afloat despite the tsunami of excess – too much pain, too much work, too much stress. Life was becoming too much and I felt I was drowning.

Realising this was a breakthrough in itself. That phone call made me take stock and really look at myself and my life. However it wasn't until after I met a neurosurgeon who explained the brain surgery recommended for my condition that the wheels of change were really set in motion. I knew I didn't want surgery to be part of my future.

I knew I couldn't change my destination overnight but I needed to change direction and explore calmer waters. At that stage I had no idea of, and I really wasn't prepared for, the voyage of discovery and transformation I was about to embark on, guided only by my desire and faith in a higher power that I could manage my pain and achieve greater health, happiness and overall wellness and balance.

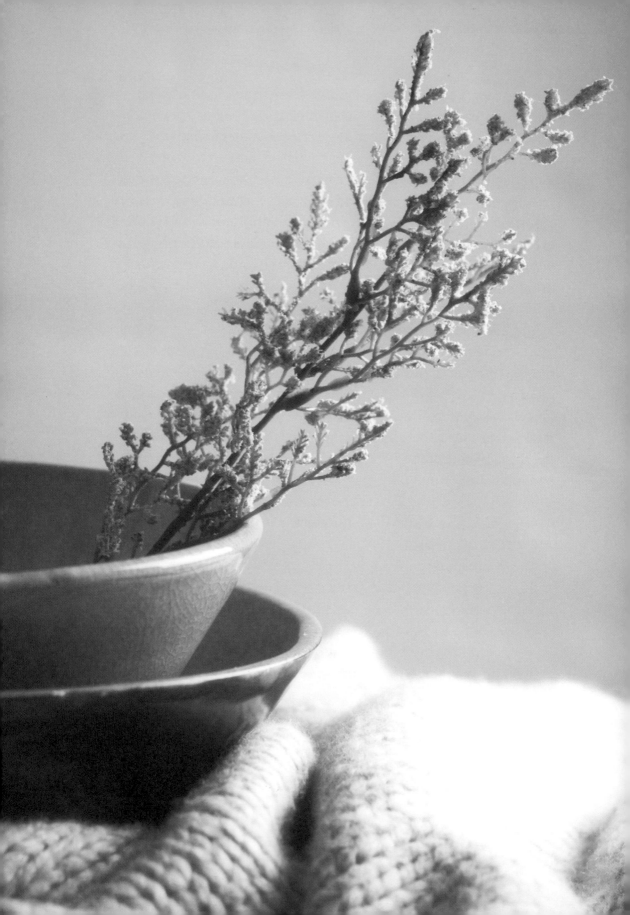

In January 2014 I took three months' leave from TV3 and began a much more important daily job – self-care. I had spent my whole working career being dedicated and determined, achieving and completing many goals with real passion. So I decided to apply those same qualities to the well-being of my mind, body and soul. It wasn't all calm waters – change represents uncertainty, whether it's planned or unplanned, and it can be very uncomfortable. Now, when I speak at events and meet other pain sufferers – whether their pain is emotional or physical – I suggest they do what I did and embrace that unease, using it to re-examine their lives and consider what direction really matters most. For me, it was my health.

My advice is to listen to the inner you and make a shift – be willing to let go of what no longer serves you. Situations, relationships, jobs, hobbies and places all have expiry dates. If something no longer feels good don't be afraid to get rid of it. Sometimes by letting go we set ourselves free to explore and manifest brilliant new possibilities. This book is designed to help you do that, to focus on your goals, to develop, step by step, changes in your life that will help you reach those goals and transform your life and, I hope, overcome the pain, whatever its source. At the end of each section I have included extracts from my own personal journal so you can see how journaling helped me in each of the areas I've outlined.

As part of my journey I have trained as a clinical hypnotherapist and have designed specific recordings that will help you access both relaxation and your inner self to aid your progress. Use these as much or as little as you need to – if you've never listened to anything like this before, let this be your first step to change. It will take one minute of your life and will greatly enhance the benefits of this journal. As you turn the pages, come with me on a journey to wellness and fulfilment.

Andrea x

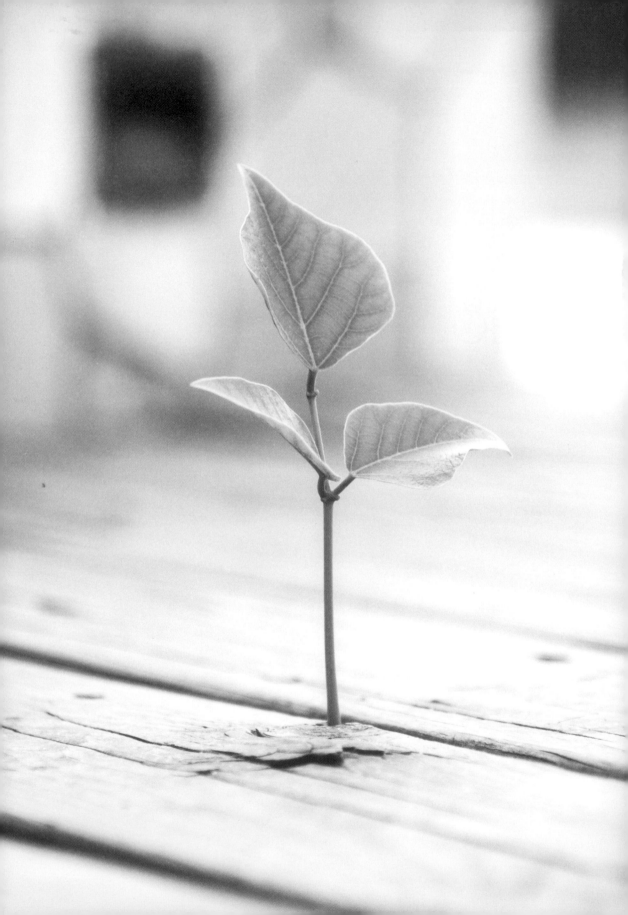

JOURNALING FOR CHANGE

'A problem shared is
a problem halved'

Do you have a dream about harvesting a new future but don't know where to begin? A journal is the perfect place to manifest change and is an excellent place for you to start.

Through using this journal you will see yourself grow into a new, stronger you over time. I have been journaling for many years and I cannot explain the phenomenon of my life goals journal except to say this: it works. There is plenty of evidence that writing down your feelings produces positive therapeutic effects on your overall health, and this journal can help you harness that, giving you space you to write your own main goals for the year ahead plus how you are feeling on a week-to-week basis. **Nothing changes unless *you* do**, so to truly experience change in your life you need to stick to the practice of journaling and make it your intention to write every day.

Think about this journey like planting a new garden; decide now which seeds of change you want to grow. Start by choosing twelve easy goals or dreams you want to manifest or harvest over the next year: focus on one each month, follow the plan of journaling weekly and do the work!

Making a commitment to complete the tasks and enjoy the process of growing will result in a new, stronger, more authentic you. When you see the little green shoots of change in your own life appear it will be so exciting – you might have to dig deep to root out any old habits that need to be replaced with new ones, but this journal work will be the genesis of a **new you**.

Better still, what begins to bloom in this journal will add boundless colour and creativity to your life and the seeds will continue to grow every year. Once you learn how to use these tools, you will have them for life and can keep using them.

In this journal, you can jot down your goals for the year ahead and easily review them, seeing how you are feeling as each month passes. Using the accompanying monthly hypnosis relaxation, you can focus on your wellness in the alpha-relaxation state of mind – the state where you are totally relaxed and open to growth and change – and this will truly solidify your new goals in your psyche.

Writing your intention to live well will anchor it in place – you can't edit what isn't written, and you cannot read over empty pages, so even if you think your writing isn't very good, keep going. You are the only person who will see this book so never worry about being judged for its contents.

HOW TO USE THIS JOURNAL

Spaces have been left throughout each chapter for you to fill in, or you can start your own separate journal and use this book as inspiration. This is your sacred space to write your personal manifesto for the life you want to create. Don't let anyone else influence what you want to achieve or what you write in this journal.

* **Be honest, be truthful, be yourself, be consistent and be willing to allow change to manifest.** Share your deepest thoughts, dreams, ideas and true emotions, no matter how weird or self-indulgent they might seem; this journal is for you, no one else, so leave judgement outside these pages. You might be as surprised as me! By opening up about my true feelings about my health and my desire to be well, wonderful new opportunities opened up for me. I believe they will for you too.

* **Enjoy writing your journal**. It is very cathartic – think of it as personal therapy. I was so surprised by how much I learned about myself in the process, how I found my authentic self and how powerful that was.

* **Inspired space.** These are little inspirational prompt boxes for you to fill in. You can write just one word or a short phrase to describe your present thoughts. For example, what are you feeling right now as you read this journal?

WHEN SHOULD YOU USE THIS JOURNAL?

In order to make writing about your journey a habit, it helps to write at a specific time each day. Everyone has different demands on their time and different schedules but it is important to allocate time with your journal, 'me time', and establish that as part of your routine.

An ideal time to write in your journal is first thing in the morning, as soon as you wake up. This can help you set the tone for the day and get into a mindset aligned with your wellness intentions. But choose a time that works for you – perhaps just before bed is better, or during your coffee break?

Even when you don't have time to write, you can still take a few moments to review your goals and wellness journey. And even when you are out and about, you can take time to listen to the monthly relaxations – listen to them on your phone if you are on the bus on your way to work or waiting in the car while collecting children from school. Ensure you take a moment out of your busy day to centre yourself – this will bring you closer to your sacred place of wellness.

Self-hypnosis

After my diagnosis of Chiari malformation 1 in December 2013, I explored everything I could about the condition. In simple terms it is a neurological disorder where part of the brain, the cerebellum (or more specifically the cerebellar tonsils), descends out of the skull into the spinal area. This results in compression of parts of the brain and spinal cord and disrupts the normal flow of cerebrospinal fluid. There was a strong chance that this rare malformation could be the underlying cause of my lifelong pain.

I felt that if I had something wrong with my brain, I should start looking for a solution from within, rather than invasive surgery or additional drugs, as my first option.

I was inspired by stories of spontaneous remission and 'miraculous' healing; I researched the phenomenon of the placebo effect – could our brains be so powerful that we can convince ourselves to recover from an illness by taking a harmless, inert substance like a sugar pill? Could the answer to my pain relief be somehow within my own mind?

The phrase 'being of two minds' summarises the mental battle that lay ahead. My conscious day-to-day mind was screaming at me that I had a diagnosis of a brain problem and chronic pain that wasn't going away. Coming to terms with this was a huge issue.

I had to remind myself that studies show that we use only a small percentage of our conscious mind for logic and reasoning. The real work is done in the subconscious mind, the part responsible for all of your involuntary actions. I knew that in order to harness the power of my mind to achieve my goals, I needed to understand how both the conscious and the subconscious mind work together and take advantage of their combined power. According to Dr Emmanuel Donchin, Director of the Laboratory for Cognitive Psychophysiology at the University of Illinois: 'An enormous portion of cognitive activity is non-conscious. Figuratively speaking, it could be 99 percent; we probably will never know precisely how much is outside awareness.'

So if the conscious part of my brain was merely the captain of the ship shouting out the orders, the main action was taking place deep down in the engine room – in the subconscious and the deeper unconscious. Captain Conscious may be in charge of the ship and giving the orders, but it's the crew that actually guides the ship, so I needed to find a new map and begin a new path of exploration.

I spent days writing out and repeating affirmations about my ability to heal. I relaxed my mind, body and spirit in meditation and visualised myself pain free.

I was doing well, but the rough seas of the mind are a lot harder to sail than I had expected and I needed help. I sought advice from an expert hypnotherapist and began weekly hypnosis sessions. Over time I travelled into the deep, dark underbelly of my unconscious.

It really surprised me to learn our subconscious mind is always working and does not appear to be limited in any way. Many believe that one of its functions is to attract outcomes and circumstances into our lives according to our predominant thought patterns. Our subconscious mind will act upon any request or instruction we give it.

Any thought that is repeated over and over can leave an imprint within the subconscious. Crucially, the subconscious mind cannot distinguish between what is real and what is imagined. This is why, when you watch a scary movie, for a few seconds while the conscious mind is chilling out in the movie 'zone', the subconscious can kick in and truly believe that blood is running down the walls of a house in Amityville. We've all been there – we get a momentary fright before our conscious mind takes over to reassure us that it is all just make-believe.

Hypnosis is the perfect vehicle to enter that trance-like state where your conscious mind can rest and allow the subconscious mind to take over and truly believe the new suggestions and beliefs we are implanting.

Visualisations, affirmations, intentions and repeated images, therefore, can have a hugely powerful effect on our lives. By doing these exercises we are creating positive images which the subconscious then acts upon.

For me hypnosis was a great success: I had seen benefits such as weight loss, reduction of my meditation and overall I was achieving my goals easier and quicker. So after months of being the client I decided to study to become the master. With no other motivation than my own healing, I started a course in clinical hypnotherapy with a wonderful teacher, Niamh Flynn at the Galway Clinic. At the end of 2014 I passed my exams and became a certified clinical hypnotherapist.

At this point I really began to dive deep into the ocean of my mind. One of the biggest breakthroughs for me was erasing the word 'pain' from my daily dialogue – I replaced it with the word 'sensations'. This one change had a hugely positive effect on me. Changing the language of pain and removing the word 'pain' from my day-to-day life rejuvenated me.

There is mounting evidence to support the idea that the mind has a role in affecting our health and physiology and in the treatment and management of chronic pain.

Research carried out in a 2000 study (by psychologists Steven Lynn, Irving Kirsch, Arreed Barabasz, Etzel Cardeña and David Patterson) revealed that one of the key benefits associated with hypnosis is the ability to alter the psychological components of the experience of pain which may then have an effect on even severe pain.

For me, I wanted to decrease my sensitivity to pain – known as hypno-analgesia. Over time, the new hypnosis technique and methods that I used daily changed my relationship with my chronic illness.

I truly believe everyone can have success if they can harness the mind–body connection.

I was fuelled by my faith in myself to be well, my positive expectation that I would have success and my desire to keep going. Like any form of training, daily hypnosis requires commitment and I flexed my mental healing muscles every day until I could really see and, most importantly, feel the benefits.

I have now adapted my hypnosis relaxations and use them in all areas of my life: stress reduction, sleeping habits, weight loss, and even getting new jobs and manifesting exciting opportunities. I believe they are the foundation of all the wonderful abundance in my life.

Using my life goals journal and healing relaxations to harness the power of the alpha state of mind go hand in hand for me. I feel they are the seeds of my success and that they can be for you too.

USING THE SELF-HYPNOSIS RELAXATIONS ON MY WEBSITE

Using the self-hypnosis relaxations in the 'My Life Goals Journal' section of my website, www.andreahayes.ie, is easy and very effective. It is also free and you can do it as often as you need at a time that suits your schedule and lifestyle.

Hypnotherapeutic approaches have been shown to be very effective in helping people to change their thought processes and, eventually, behaviours; this can assist us in feeling more self-confident and focused on achieving our intentions and goals.

Hypnosis works by first achieving a state of highly focused attention with heightened suggestibility.

The best brainwave state of mind for hypnosis is the alpha state. There are four brainwave states: beta, alpha, theta and delta. Beta is the normal conscious state we are in every day; alpha is a relaxed, drowsy state; theta is the light sleep state or deep meditative state; and delta is the deep sleep or coma state.

Proven benefits of hypnosis and deep meditative relaxation include increased focus, reduced anxiety, increased creativity, reduced stress, increased memory, reduced pain, increased compassion, reduced depression and increased productivity. Hypnosis cultivates willpower, builds focus and concentration, boosts cognitive function, reduces depression and physically changes the brain, aiding sleep, building self-knowledge, helping in relationship satisfaction, improving empathy and promoting emotional wellness.

To really help your new goals become your reality, use the power of your mind and the twelve themed hypnosis relaxations that accompany your journal.

Tips on how to achieve great change

1. Give achieving your goals and intentions a high priority. Plan to use self-hypnosis on a daily basis and you will start to see results.

2. Write your thoughts, feelings, intentions and goals down in your journal. Each month we have a theme to work on – if you have other intentions, simply clarify what you want to work on and be specific. Make sure you set intentions that are achievable. If they are long-term goals, it may be helpful to break them down into manageable steps and give them a specific time frame – for example, four weeks.

3. During each relaxation there is a time for self-reflection and visualisation. Formulate your hypnotic intentions and goals and write them down. Make sure you really believe them to be true for you – write out a number of intentions for the goal you are working on.

4. Remember, seeing is believing. Decide on the imagery you plan to use. If your aim is to relax, picture a pleasant scene like a beach or a forest on a warm summer's day.

5. Repetition is central to success. Remember to use your short relaxation daily: the most effective time to use it is upon waking and just before you go to sleep at night. It can also be used throughout the day as an effective relaxation tool to alleviate stress.

HOW TO REACH YOUR ALPHA

Alpha is a lightly relaxed state, a place to begin hypnosis and visualisation.

Close your eyes and relax. With every deep breath you take you'll deepen your alpha state further. It might take a little practice but you will learn to master your brainwaves and become an expert at effective self-hypnosis. It all begins with relaxation: by using the twelve audio relaxations to accompany this journal on my website you will be effectively tapping into your alpha state, preparing the subconscious mind to be programmed.

Each relaxation has embedded suggestions for the theme of the month it appears in. But you can also use your own power of visualisation to send effective messages to your subconscious mind to facilitate your desired change. Visualisations are especially effective because the subconscious mind works best with imagery.

The secret to harnessing the power of your mind is to clearly visualise the situation, the action and the feeling that you desire. Use all your senses when picturing a desired outcome. Use your senses of touch, hearing, sight and even smell.

I sometimes visualise I am at a cinema: I have a crystal clear image of my desired goal and I pretend I am watching a movie and clearly 'see' myself 'in the role', feeling how I would 'feel' when my desire became a reality.

Your life goals journal year

Over the next twelve months this journal will take you through a series of stages from self-improvement and goal setting to a place where you can play an active part in controlling your life. At each step you can see how my story progressed in extracts from my own journal. It worked for me and I believe it can work for you too.

Each month and topic has its own healing hypnosis relaxation for you to listen to. If you feel you want to skip ahead, do that – this is your journal to use in the way that best suits you. Each month the relaxation is a little longer and there are more on my website, www.andreahayes.ie, if you need them.

Think of the seeds you want to plant to change your life. Allow this journal to be a garden of successes: sow potential bounty and trust you will grow and harvest wellness and endless possibilities.

Your journal pages – make them fun!

Your journal is the place you come to be yourself and focus on yourself – make it a lovely thing that you look forward to opening. Choose images and words to enhance the changes you want to develop. Find pictures in magazines and cut out words and stick them in your journal to give you inspiration.

Sometimes all you need to begin writing is just one word. I have given you a list of positive words to use as prompts, but you have the freedom to write about anything you want. Choose a word that resonates with you or go day by day through the list and allow yourself to be inspired.

We are each unique, so there will be some words that sum up your values and goals better than others. Feel free to add your own words to create your own personal mix when you are writing your journal. Adding any of these words to the pages will help bring more vibrancy to your thoughts and feelings.

REAL Independence Romance
TRUE CREATIVITY
Wellness
AUTHENTIC L Peace
Smile Strength
Power JOY Divine
Relax calm
FEARLESS V YES
Balance Harmony GRATITUDE MIRACLE
FRIENDSHIP
ZEAL E Secure Transform
Patience Free
Appreciate
MAGNIFICENT FUN
HEALTH Values
SELF-ESTEEM

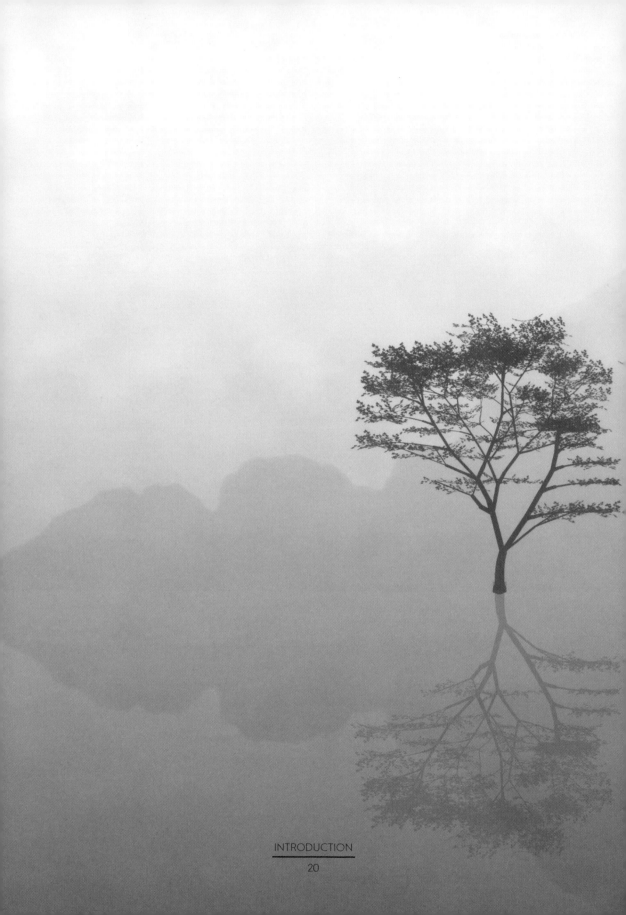

'Your mind is the garden
Your thoughts are the seeds
The harvest can either be
flowers or weeds'

– Variant of the William Wordsworth poem

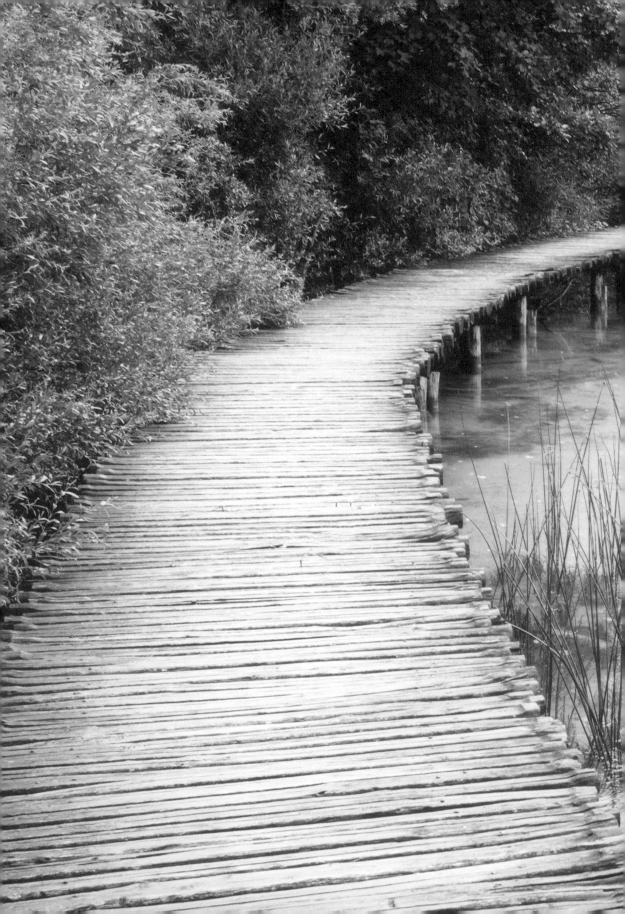

MONTH 1

Being the True You and Goal Setting

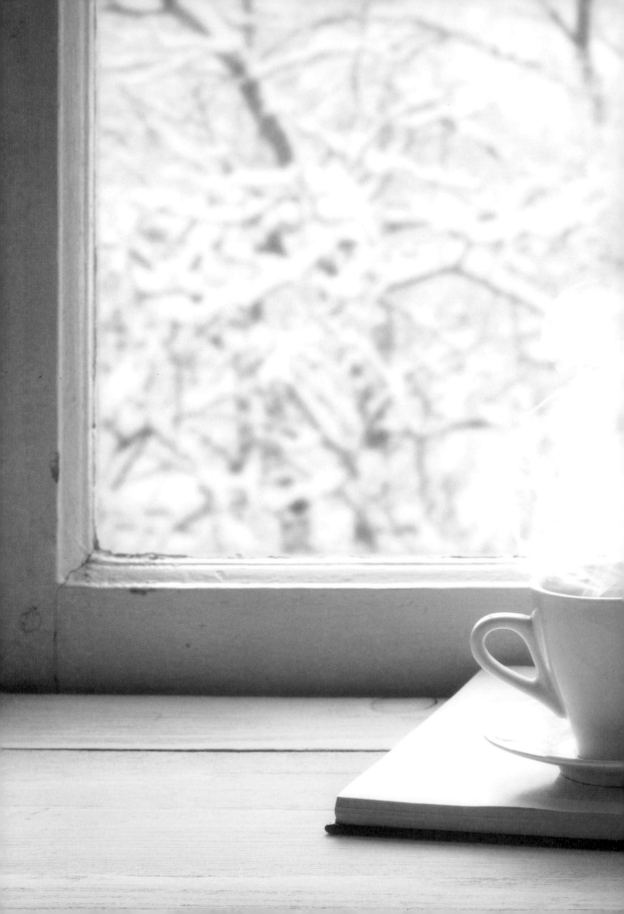

'Be a first rate version of yourself, not a second rate version of someone else'

– Judy Garland

As you start this journey make the intention now to **be true to the real you**. You are wonderfully unique and bring something special into the world. You cannot be copied. Now is the time to embrace your authentic self and allow this process of development to unfold.

When I began my journey to wellness I really struggled with this starting point – with becoming my true self. I had to ask what that meant. It might seem self-explanatory – you are who you are; you wake up and live your life and are you.

However, living with pain, this wasn't true for me. I was living a lie, pretending everything was OK. I was putting on a mask to the world and not really living a life that was in tune with my authentic self or who I was created to truly be.

I wasn't being honest, I wasn't even happy and I wasn't embracing all the different parts of my personality that make me uniquely 'me'. I was living like a fictional character in many ways and living in a way I felt the world thought I should be. I was allowing other people's perceptions to colour my actions.

> Ask yourself now if you are aware of the two versions of your 'self' that are co-existing.
>
> Are you suppressing your genuine self, your creativity and your authenticity, without even being aware that you are doing so?

Becoming authentic is an individual mission, since each person is truly unique – this is why honesty and genuine self-awareness are central to the process of real change.

You now have this journal in your hand and you are beginning a new journey: many fresh ideas about your true self and your path in life will manifest. This new, stronger you may surprise or threaten others, as they may not have the same vision, motivation or commitment that you have to welcome change into your life.

Be aware now that this is your unique life goals journey – don't allow other people's ideas to send you off course. Stay on your path and trust you are taking steps day by day to a new, exciting destination that will bring you true joy and freedom from old patterns and ingrained limitations.

Think back on your life and consider your upbringing, the values and learned patterns of behaviours you have adopted since childhood. Maybe you have been living your life with a notion that you must achieve certain things? Maybe you felt you should have a certain job, a certain relationship, live in a certain place or act a certain way in order to be respected and validated? Maybe you were told you could *not* be a certain type of person or achieve a particular thing? If we reflect on past choices in our lives it can help us really define if we are being true to whom we are at our deepest core level.

> Do you want to change some of those core ideas and beliefs? To release yourself from what other people think so you can live your life as the true you? This is the place to start.

Who Are You?

When you're asked, 'Who are you?' what is your answer?

It is very easy to say 'I am a mother', 'I am a teacher', 'I am a parent', 'I am a good person' – but who are you? Perhaps you are all these things?

Or do you find yourself saying 'I am sick and tired of work' or 'I am always the one who ends up doing all the work' or 'I am always being treated badly by people'?

What you attach **I am** to is very powerful in your subconscious belief system, as you are literally affirming to yourself what you believe to be true for yourself at this moment.

Make a list right now and ask yourself, who am I?

Become aware of your **I am** answers – remember you are the one filling in the blanks and telling your subconscious mind what your reality is.

WHO AM I?

I am ...

....

....

....

....

....

....

....

....

Is your answer more about what you do or where you see yourself in society than about who you really are in life?

Sometimes it is a very challenging question to answer. If you can't answer who you are, maybe it is because you don't know, or have simply lost sight of your true self? In today's world, when we are constantly bombarded with images of how we should be, how we should act and how we should think, it is important to understand who you really are.

After my diagnosis, I needed to take time out to begin to find myself again and truly reassess my life, my values and who I wanted to be. I needed to stop so I could understand how to be true to my core. I also decided that I would remove the word *should* from my life, and replace it with *could* – I could do whatever I wanted, which gave me the power to make a choice. We all have the power to choose to make changes in our lives. If you want to allow your true self to be seen then now is the time for you to make long-term plans and set new goals for a positive, successful future.

'With every act of self care your authentic self gets stronger, and the critical, fearful mind gets weaker. Every act of self care is a powerful declaration: I am on my side; each day I am more and more on my side'

– Susan Weiss Berry

TRY THIS EXERCISE

Ask yourself now, what do you really want in life?

....

....

....

....

....

....

....

....

....

For me it was simple: I wanted more balance. I was working so much, all my relationships began to suffer. I wanted to put my health and wellness first, so I decided to **make me the priority**. I became conscious of the choices I was making: my new decisions needed to reflect my goal of changing the way I was living my life.

MY ANSWERS

1. Include meditation and relaxation in my daily routine
2. Eat a healthier diet and feel fitter
3. Create more time for myself, my family and my friends
4. Choose work that inspires and excites me
5. Reduce my medication

It's not always easy to know what you want, but the better the understanding you have of what you truly want for the future, the better the grasp you'll get on your true self. Make a list of your goals – they can be aspirational at first, but think about what would make you happy.

DECIDE FOR YOURSELF

This time next year I want to be ...

1. ....

....

2. ....

....

3. ....

....

4. ....

....

5. ....

....

In my case, when I embarked on my journal writing it was all about my wellness and living as well as I could, in my mind, body and inner spirit. For me this came down to really **reassessing** my values and goals and **prioritising** what was most important. You need to ask yourself what your goals are for the next year and beyond.

Do you want to live a healthier life? Do you want to retire? Get married? Do you want to change career? Be rich? Live in a different country? Write a book? Learn a new skill? Run a marathon?

Understanding and becoming the true you will result in all sorts of benefits. Remember, what you attach I AM to is powerful.

I AM:

HAPPINESS,
CONFIDENCE, PEACE,
JOY, HONESTY,
LOVE, SATISFACTION,
RESILIENCE,
TRUTHFULNESS,
FULFILMENT,
CONTENTMENT,
SELF-AWARENESS,
KINDNESS, ACCEPTANCE,
COURAGEOUSNESS,
BEAUTY.

MAKE YOUR OWN LIST

I am:

I realised I hadn't actually given much thought to how I wanted my life to unfold and that's why I had lost touch with my true self.

When was the last time you took some time to think long and hard about your goals? Are these goals the same as they were ten years ago? Probably not. We all change as our lives and circumstances change so every year we should take time out to re-evaluate our lives and behaviour and make sure we are making the right choices to bring our life goals to fruition.

I believe you can do this and now is the time for you to **believe in yourself** and your own ability to **change your reality** and have faith in yourself that this can happen.

TRY THIS EXERCISE

Be fearless and dare to **dream big**. Be in alignment with your life's purpose. If you do not know what you want to achieve in life ask yourself these questions.

What do I want my purpose in life to be?

How would I like to be remembered?

What makes me happiest in life?

How can I make a contribution to help others?

....

....

....

Check back over the answers written here every month or so – think about whether you are closer to achieving them. Even baby steps become strides in time.

This journal is about setting goals and achieving those goals: **statements of intent**. Our goals tell us what we want to achieve, how we want to change or how we want to look or act sometime in the future.

Decide each day what you want to focus on – keep that goal or idea central in your thoughts all day. Writing down our goals, and even sharing them with other people, makes it easier for our brain to accept them as reality.

> **Repetition of your intentions will make your goals more achievable: say your goals daily; write them out and carry them around with you every day!**

Your goals and intentions will be more effective if they are specific and realistic. If you wish to improve your swimming performance, it would be unrealistic to set yourself the goal of becoming a world-class swimmer – unless, of course, you are already on the Olympic team.

SMART PLAN
Setting SMART goals

Think about using the **SMART** system – SMART is an acronym designed to help you set objectives (often attributed to Peter Drucker's management-by-objectives concept). It is ideal for setting personal goals.

S Simple specific goal

M Measurable

A Achievable

R Realistic

T Tense

(I add an extra PLAN)

P Positive feeling

L Love

A Action

N No excuses

What's your SMART PLAN? For example, if you want to lose weight, this is how you would apply this method.

SIMPLE

– *I want to lose weight.*
(A simple and specific goal)

MEASURABLE

– *I want to lose* one stone *in weight.*
(You can measure and track your weight loss)

ACHIEVABLE

– *I want to lose one stone in weight* in six months.
(Here you are giving yourself a time frame to achieve your goal)

REALISTIC

– *I want to lose one stone in weight in six months* by eating healthily and exercising three times a week.
(Here you are giving yourself a realistic way to help you achieve your goal)

TENSE (PRESENT TENSE)

– *I want to lose one stone in weight in six months by eating healthily and exercising three times a week,* beginning today until June.
(You are setting a present-day deadline to achieve your goal – it is beginning *now*, not in the future)

POSITIVE FEELING

– *I want to lose one stone in weight in six months by eating healthily and exercising three times a week, beginning today until June.* I will feel positive health benefits with my new lifestyle.
(This encourages you to attach positive benefits to achieving your goal, which will go a long way to helping you achieve it)

LOVE

– I want to lose one stone in weight in six months by eating healthily and exercising three times a week, beginning today until June. I will feel positive health benefits with my new lifestyle. By achieving this goal it will be an act of self-love.

(Prioritising your goal and making time to achieve it is an act of self-love that will bring you well-being and great happiness)

ACTION

– I want to lose one stone in weight in six months by eating healthily and exercising three times a week, beginning today until June. I will feel positive health benefits with my new lifestyle. By achieving this goal it will be an act of self-love. I will get up early to walk to work and prepare and plan my dinners every Sunday for the week ahead and measure my weight loss every week.

(Here you are stating what specific steps you need to take to achieve your goal and including a day for review and forward planning)

NO EXCUSES

– I want to lose one stone in weight in six months by eating healthily and exercising three times a week, beginning today until June. I will feel positive health benefits with my new lifestyle. By achieving this goal it will be an act of self-love. I will get up early to walk to work and prepare and plan my dinners every Sunday for the week ahead and measure my weight loss every week. I will be disciplined and consistent until I reach my goal.

(You are taking personal accountability for your actions and decisions so you make every effort to achieve your goal)

SAY IT AS IF YOU MEAN IT.

WRITE IT AS IF YOU BELIEVE IT.

VISUALISE IT AS IF IT HAS ALREADY BECOME A REALITY.

Road map to achieving your goals

MY GOALS

Using your answers from the previous exercises as inspiration, write down twelve goals you would like to work on for the duration of this journal.

1. ....

....

2. ....

....

3. ....

....

4. ....

....

5. ....

....

6. ....

....

7. ....

....

8. ....

....

9. ....

....

10. ....

....

11. ....

....

12. ....

Why not choose a goal and, using the **SMART PLAN** method, see how you can apply the principles and make it a reality?

Simple goal
....

Measurable
....

Achievable
....

Realistic
....

Tense
....

Positive feeling
....

Love
....

Action
....

No Excuses
....

'If you wish to move mountains tomorrow, you must start by lifting stones today'

– African Proverb

Now that you have goals to focus on, try this.

DARE OF THE DAY

Start each day by looking into the mirror and repeating your goal for the day.

DARE OF THE WEEK

Share your goal with an accountability buddy! As long as the goal is not too personal or confidential in nature, telling a trusted friend about it will make you more accountable and more likely to achieve your goal. Plus, the support will help you to stay focused.

OUR ACCOUNTABILITY BUDDY

It is important to consider carefully who might fulfill the role of accountability buddy. This is someone who will help you keep on track – it needs to be someone you can trust, who does not judge you or seek to influence you, someone who knows you for you. There is no need to share everything with your buddy, no need to explain that you are journaling. Their role is to give you positive encouragement and to see how far you have come on your journey. If you don't have a suitable friend, don't worry – perhaps make that one of your goals?

If you share your dream with someone else, like a friend or family member, not only will you get support from him or her but also it is more likely that you will achieve your goals because suddenly you are accountable to someone other than just yourself.

In the same way, if you begin a course you are accountable to the lecturer and you have to pass exams, or if you have specific health goals and work with a trainer you are accountable to someone who shares your dream and will help you stay on track.

* Tell someone what you plan to do and ask him or her to check in with you weekly or monthly.

* Seek out like-minded people who will encourage you to stay on track.

* Reward yourself for achieving your milestones.

DARE OF THE MONTH

Take time this month to achieve one of the goals on your list.

HOW ARE YOU FEELING RIGHT NOW?

HOW GOAL SETTING HELPED ME:
extract from my journal

I am feeling very grateful today for my focus and commitment to my new health goals and lifestyle choices. I visited my GP this morning and we spoke about reducing my medication during the three months that I have decided to take off work. We have a plan of action with goals that I feel are achievable and I know they will be bringing me closer to being more in charge of my health and well-being.

I wanted to reduce my medication a bit quicker than she suggested, but I know from experience she is right and it needs to be done slowly. There are no quick fixes – all change takes time and needs proper planning and preparation, and her advice about my medication-reduction goals made me think a lot about my life goals in general. While I have taken time off to focus solely on my wellness, maybe this is really about looking at all areas of my life, not just my health? The work I want to do, the way I live my life, the food I eat – really, everything. When I went out for my walk I tried to focus fully on what I wanted to achieve.

I started the year calling it my 'soul and healing diet year'. A 'diet' seemed like an odd way of looking at it, but when I thought about it, it seemed perfect. After Christmas we are bombarded with 'New Year, New You' diet plans and maybe subliminally that affected me. But I have to eliminate some things – as with any 'diet', certain things are not good for you, certainly not healthy. I have to change my life and introduce good systems and practices. And as with any diet, I have fallen off the wagon – I didn't do my daily stretches relaxation today – but writing down my feelings, all those things I agreed with myself I would do, helps me see that one fail isn't a disaster. Tomorrow I will be able to do better.

Instead of blaming my failure on the pain, which I had been doing, I'm really taking responsibility, and looking back, that's been one of my biggest lessons in recent weeks. I have the power to change – it's my relationship with 'me, myself and I' that is the key to any major changes I want to achieve.

I want to really consider what it is I want in life.

The first thing is more balance – I want to focus on my health and family for these three months and put the same commitment and dedication I put into my work goals into my new health goals. This is my priority right now and I feel good about making it my focus and giving it my attention. I am forever reading sayings that suggest putting yourself first isn't an act of selfishness but an act of great kindness to oneself, and maybe it is time for me to give myself some time. My job for the next few months is **me** – project me!

I'm finding thinking about myself in more detail very enlightening. I asked myself not only what do I really want but also what is my life's mission. Immediately I thought of my daughter Brooke and being the perfect mum to her, but I was also reminded about how much enjoyment I used to get from being involved in projects that I am passionate about. So I have decided I want to commit some of my time to doing more charity work locally.

I'm going to take note of all the things I do daily or weekly that bring me happiness – I want to do more of what makes me happy and less of what causes me stress and strain. Even just writing that now is powerful, as I am acknowledging that my happiness is important. I am taking stock and really starting to become mindful of how I am feeling and asking myself, is this making me happy? It has been wonderful already to see that little things like walking Dash actually make me a little happier. It is like I'm reframing my mind – instead of feeling that I have to walk the dog, I say to myself: 'I know this will fill me with joy and truly isn't it a blessing that my legs and body are well enough for me to walk today.' Listing my thinking on things has changed something in me already.

'The secret of change is to focus all of your energy, not on fighting the old, but building the new'

– Socrates

MONTHLY REVIEW

- ▸ This month's hypnosis relaxation will help you to ground yourself and develop your daily goals.

- ▸ Use the free journal pages to write down your own personal entries and remember to be mindful of this month's theme of being the true you and setting new goals for the months ahead.

- ▸ Make it your intention to listen to your daily hypnosis relaxation on my website and try to write about how you find the experience.

- ▸ Write honestly and consistently, and remember nothing you write is wrong: there is no judgement in your journal so be true to your feelings and be free!

PROMPTS

Name the things you do that make you feel good:

_____

_____

_____

_____

_____

_____

_____

_____

_____

What is your life plan?

Are there parts of yourself you hide from others?

My Journal

'*My aim is to put down on paper what I see and what I feel in the best and simplest way.*'

– Ernest Hemingway

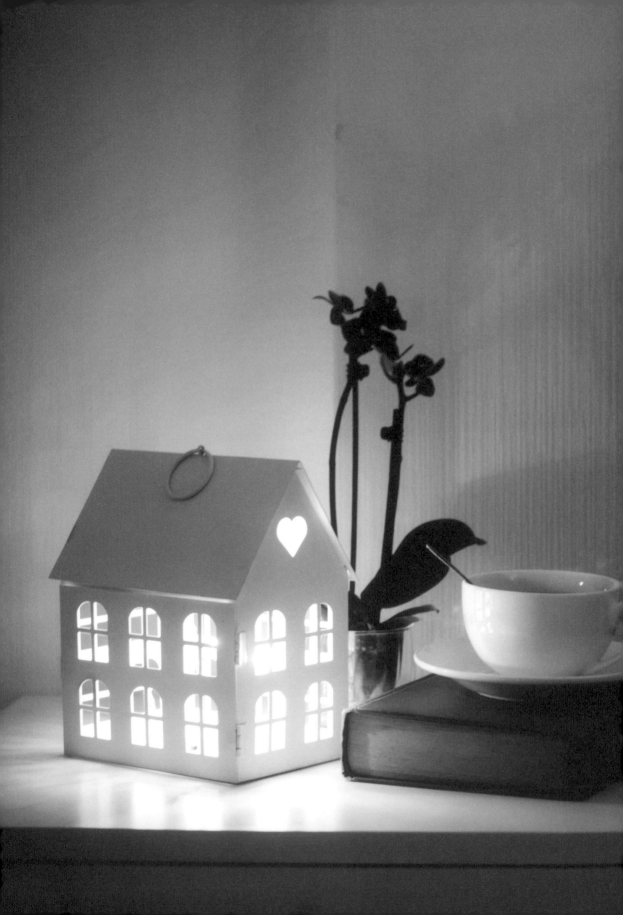

MONTH 2

Love and self-care

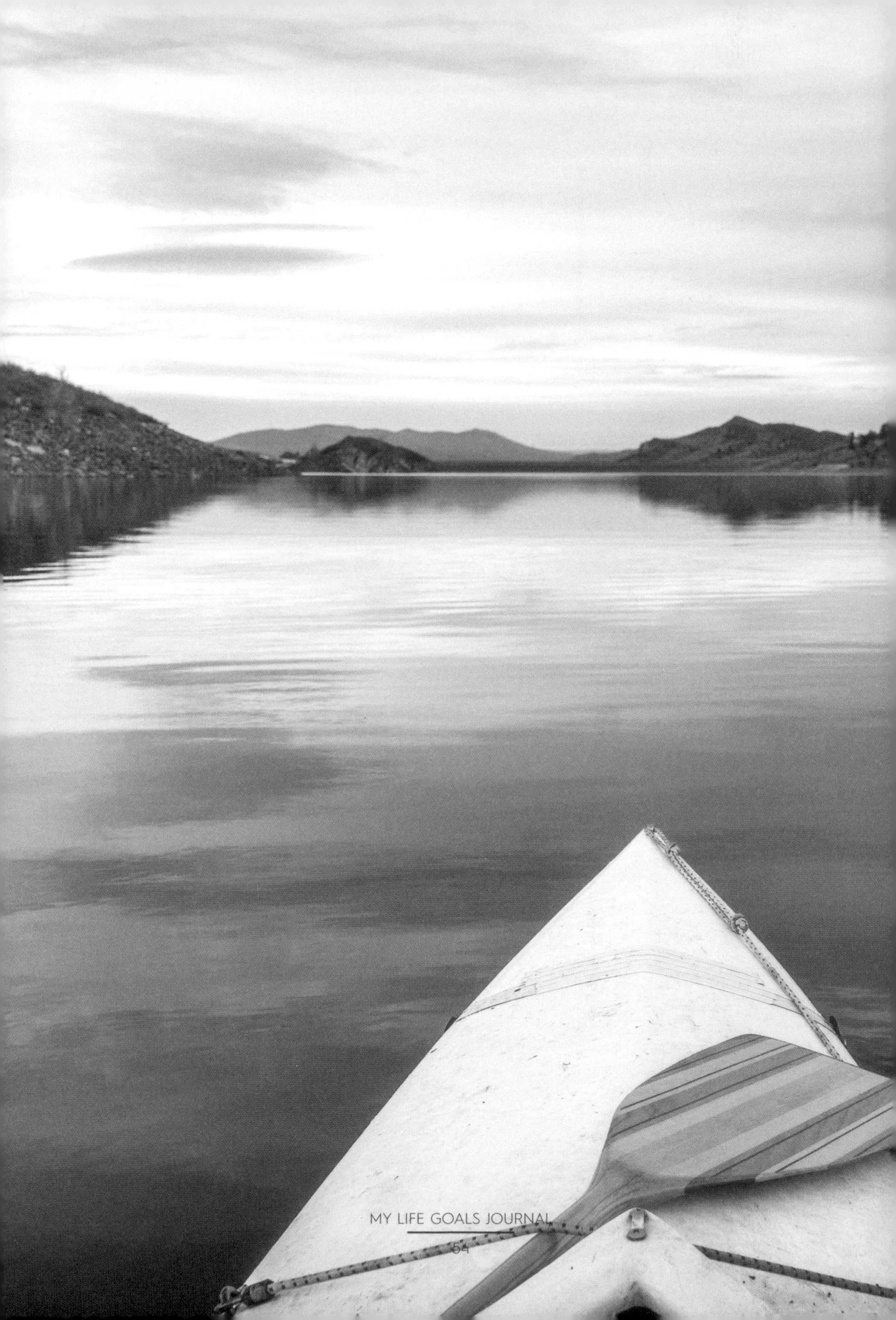

'To thine own self be true'

– William Shakespeare

Begin this month with an expectation of love for everything in your life. If I asked you to name all the things you **love** in your world, how long would it take you to say yourself? This week start every day by saying to yourself **I love you**!

Our lives can get very hectic and sometimes it feels like our world is a busy crossroads, with demands on our time constantly pulling our energy in different directions. It is very easy to always be giving and allowing your engine to almost run on empty.

We find ourselves caring for our families, our friends, our work, our homes, our neighbours – and in the midst of all these concerns and activities, what happens? We totally forget about looking after the most important person – our self.

How often have you said, 'I have so much to do!'?

Think about how much you are doing for yourself. After all, how are you going to give to others if you are not looking after you first?

I was totally at odds with my life and even with my body because I felt it somehow had let me down. I was crippled with pain daily and that is very difficult to overcome. Instead of feeling love for the wonderful gift of life, I was focusing on all the negatives in my life – life was a chore from the moment I got out of bed until I ended the day, and all the while I had the additional burden of constant pain.

'I can handle this,' I told myself. 'I'll be fine.'

And I did seem fine. But my desire to please and be all things to all people was choking me – I felt like I couldn't breathe. I often would keep going and keep giving – to work and to everything and everyone else around me – until I came home and simply collapsed. In my worst moments, I had to take a couple of weeks off work and normal life to recuperate. During this time I lost my momentum, money and confidence, so I realised I needed to **stop** this frenzied routine and get my work, life and 'me' time in balance. I enjoyed being seen as a brilliant woman who could do it all, the type of person my family and friends often called on for help in matters professional and otherwise, but I needed to be honest with myself and accept I was barely surviving.

I had read studies that suggested that not taking care of ourselves is unhealthy for those who depend upon us, and I had a daughter and family to think about, as well as my own physical and mental health, so I started to practise self-love and try to **love** myself.

Don't be fooled: loving yourself isn't being self-centred or self-obsessed – it is quite the opposite, actually. It means putting effort into your self-care. This might sound easy but it takes a lot of daily commitment and focused attention to put yourself first for a change.

So why is it hard for many of us to do things for ourselves before we do so much for others? Maybe it is how we were brought up – we think looking after ourselves is being selfish – but as the old saying goes, you need to love yourself and be yourself one hundred per cent before you can love someone else.

DO YOU LOVE YOURSELF?

'Happiness is not something ready made. It comes from your own actions'

– Dalai Lama

Here are some ways to start taking care of **you**.

1. Change your language

Loving yourself fully and completely has a lot to do with the language you use about yourself. Use words to describe yourself that are **positive** and **loving**. Notice today how many times you say negative things about yourself and make an effort to stop.

Switch the words 'I should' to 'I could' or 'I would like to'. 'Should' limits your choices and immediately puts pressure on you. It is simply self-inflicted stress that you don't need. For example, instead of saying 'I should stay late at work to finish this project,' try 'I would like to clear my desk before tomorrow so I could stay on an extra hour tonight and get this done.'

Learn to say no. If you've been asked to do something or feel like you 'should' do something, ask yourself, is it something I really want to do? Learn to say **no** to things that are not what you want. It is important to say no to people and activities that drain you or fill you with negative energy. If you find it very hard to say no, instead of committing to things try saying, 'Let me get back to you on that' – it gives you time to really consider if you want to say **yes**.

2. Start to put yourself first in all your relationships

IN LOVE

Remember to **love yourself first** and keep your unique individuality alive. You deserve and need as much of your own attention as your partner does, so instead of always thinking of your partner first, remember you will be a better partner if you give yourself time for you. When you feel happy you will make the people around you happy.

AT WORK

Are you a people pleaser? Do you like to keep the peace even if it means doing more than your share of the work load? It is an act of self-love to apply some **boundaries** to your work. By setting reasonable and fair expectations at work, you can relieve the unnecessary guilt of not being able to please everyone all the time.

WITH FRIENDS

Put yourself first by focusing on friendships that stem naturally from a place of **joy** and **compatibility**. When you're surrounded by people who are similar to you, and who are equally kind and loving, you no longer need to sacrifice yourself to make the friendships work.

3. Get to know yourself with some 'me' time in your calendar

We can all lose touch with who we are and we can forget the simple pleasures that make us happy. By setting a small amount of time aside each day to get in touch with yourself you can easily re-evaluate how your day went. Think about:

1. Did I enjoy what I did today?
2. Am I looking forward to anything tomorrow?
3. Am I being true to myself and my goals?
4. Did I make time for me today?

- Don't be afraid to ask yourself what makes you happy.
- Set aside 'me' time each week to do at least one thing that you know will have the biggest impact on your personal happiness.
- You know the feeling you get when something isn't right?
- Make time to listen to that inner voice and **pause** for that time to **reflect** on what your mind and body needs.

4. Don't be afraid to ask for help

A big act of self-love is accepting that you cannot do everything alone and sometimes it is OK to ask for help – in fact, it can be essential. You may have been raised to believe it is a sign of weakness to look for assistance and you like to hide your flaws and imperfections. Or maybe you feel that by asking for help you are going to be a burden on others. But, trust me, the people who love you will be only too happy to help and there is no shame asking for it every now and then.

Make it your intention this month to **fall in love with yourself**. Pamper yourself. Do anything that uplifts your spirit. This can mean being with those you love, petting your dog or cat, going for a walk, sitting quietly by yourself – anything that puts you in a better-feeling place. Give yourself permission to do things that you love. If you can't think of ways to pamper yourself then we have some work to do – maybe giving yourself **time** is the first act of self-love.

'Too many people overvalue what they are not and undervalue what they are'

– Malcolm S. Forbes

TRY THIS EXERCISE

Take time now to write a list of ten things you can do that will make you smile and feel all happy inside.

1. ....
....

2. ....
....

3. ....
....

4. ....
....

5. ....
....

6. ....
....

7. ....
....

8. ....
....

9. ....
....

10. ....
....

You are hereby allowed to love yourself freely. Remember, listening to your hypnosis relaxation is the perfect way to enjoy some time for you. It will also help to lower your blood pressure and release stress, immediately creating a more harmonious environment with a greater ease and peace that will benefit not only you but also those around you.

DARE OF THE DAY

Start each day by looking into the mirror and repeating these three little words: **I love you**.

DARE OF THE WEEK

Book a date night with yourself at a lovely restaurant or go to see a show in the theatre. Get out a DVD you've always wanted to watch and plan something special for dinner. If the evenings don't work, pamper yourself and treat yourself to a 'you' day.

DARE OF THE MONTH

Practise self-love: accept and honour yourself. Take time out to be quiet and connect with who you really are. Write a letter to yourself and remind yourself of all the wonderful things you have achieved so far in life and all the brilliant and beautiful talents you possess.

PLAN A DATE NIGHT:

Note to self –
I don't have to take this
day all at once
One breath at a time
One moment at a time
One minute at a time

HOW I EMBRACED SELF-LOVE AND, FOR THE FIRST TIME, WENT ON A DATE WITH MYSELF:
extract from my journal

So in the spirit of self-love I set a date with myself today and it was actually great. I went for a drive to a beach I haven't been at for years and had a nice walk and then – bravely, in my opinion – went for a meal by myself in a lovely Italian restaurant. I just sat in the window and watched the world go by. I felt that this was time for me to relax, to savour delicious food and to take the time alone to think and enjoy the view. Another big lesson I have learned over the past months while I've been off work is to make my health my job daily, and I am feeling so proud of what I have achieved in such a short time.

For the first time ever I said **no** to work and **yes** to myself. When I was enjoying my lovely pasta today, the whole notion of saying no really hit home. I was on my date day, relaxing, and it suddenly just struck me: I had said no to work and said yes to my goal. I wanted to make my own wellness a full-time job and I have – and guess what? I am enjoying it.

As I walked back to my car today after my indulgent date alone, I was filled with a sense of pride in myself. I started this part of my own pain management in January of this year, and I can honestly say it has been life changing – many lessons are being learned and I have loved exploring my new path in life.

'Gently' is my new word, not 'pacing' anymore – my word is **gentle**. I do things in a gentle manner and treat myself gently and honestly. It's hard to focus totally on yourself but I am consciously taking time to really love myself and say to myself – often and with feeling – Andrea, I **love** you.

The act of self-love is so powerful. We are all craving love and attention and, really, that has to start with ourselves. If you cannot love yourself you will not be able to love anyone else. So I am dating myself and today's first date went very well – I can see myself doing this a lot more. That hair advert has been going around and around in my head all day: 'Because you're worth it.' All of us are worth it, and I am too.

'Love is the great
miracle cure. Loving
ourselves works
miracles in our lives'

– Louise L. Hay

MONTHLY REVIEW

▸ This month's hypnosis relaxation will help you with self-love and acceptance.

▸ How are you enjoying filling the pages of your own personal journal? Are you looking forward to exploring this month's theme of love and self-care?

▸ Make an effort to listen to your daily hypnosis relaxation on my website.

▸ Journaling in itself is an act of self-care so use the pages to cultivate love for you!

PROMPTS

The ways I already show love to myself are:

I acknowledge my self-worth and my past successes by:

I love myself for:

I feel at peace with myself because:

My Journal

'Journal writing is a voyage to the interior.'

             – Christina Baldwin

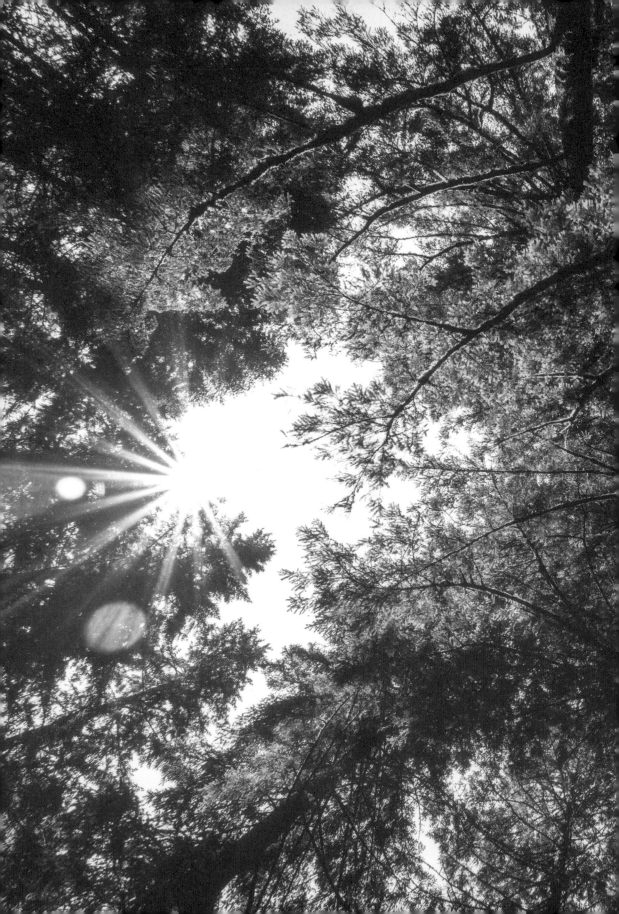

MONTH 3

Thoughts create your reality

'As you think
so shall you be'

– Dr Wayne Dyer

This month, harness the power of your amazing mind by becoming aware. Rewire your brain by changing your thoughts and learning to use the **power of positive thinking**.

What does this phrase really mean? What 'power' does thinking in a positive way really have? I am sure we'd all agree that thinking positively is a good thing, especially when we're feeling positive and life is going well. However, when you live with chronic pain and are feeling pretty crappy it is a lot harder to stay positive.

I would say I'm a pretty positive person, but I wanted to explore whether saying positive affirmations could really change how I was feeling. Could positive thinking change your brain in a physical way? I explored the science of neuroplasticity and recent research into how our brain processes pain. I was willing to do the work. Just like exercise, that work required repetition and dedication to reinforce my new mental approach to pain, and it worked for me. Every day I repeated my positive affirmations for my health goals and I truly worked each day to keep my mind focused on my intentions.

Controlling your thoughts and becoming aware of what you are thinking about can change your life.

What do your thoughts say about you?

What do they say about your life?

Do they match your vision for your life and for you in the future?

Challenge negative thought patterns by asking ...

HOW
– am I thinking about myself right now?

WHY
– am I feeling this way?

WHO
– really believes this to be true or
is it just me?

WHERE
– did this emotion or thought come from?

WHEN
– did I begin to feel like this?

WHAT
– can I do to change this thought into a
positive feeling?

'What you think
you become'

– Buddha

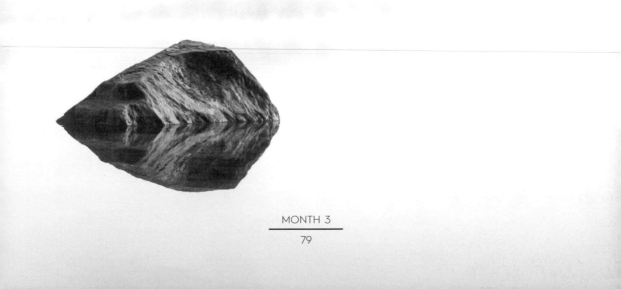

This month, take time to consciously **think** and become more aware of the good things around you and strengths that you have. Keep your thoughts positive and focused on your main goals. Take time to review those main goals that you wrote at the beginning of the book. How far have you come?

Practise **trust**: trust in yourself and replace fearful thoughts about the future with the self-knowledge that everything is unfolding perfectly for you in your world, even if it doesn't feel like that right now. Trust that everything you need will come at the right time.

Keep your thoughts about yourself positive; believe that you are capable of great things. Amazing things have manifested for me and for others from just one thought, so have faith. Believe in yourself and make your thoughts reflect this perception and you will be unstoppable.

If you haven't worked with affirmations before, consider giving it a go this month.

What is an affirmation?

An affirmation is usually a short, positive statement in the present tense. It affirms what you desire to be true or something that has already happened. Positive affirmations are used to build a positive internal dialogue. When we consistently repeat positive affirmations, we create positive subconscious thoughts and can make positive changes more quickly and automatically. We are able to create a new positive reality by replacing old and negative thinking with new and positive thoughts.

When we say an affirmation we must think consciously about our words and our thoughts and we must feel them and enjoy them. When we feel positive emotions our mind is instinctively responding to something it believes to be true and we can experience them physically. This can be very difficult at first, especially if you are in pain, but I found that repeating my affirmations kept me focused on my inner wellness goals.

TODAY
I WILL LET
MYSELF
SHINE

It can feel strange repeating an affirmation that doesn't seem right, but I found that, over time, continually repeating and writing down the affirmation definitely had a positive effect on my overall mood.

> Affirmations are a very simple way of reprogramming our thought patterns that can have a huge impact. Change your thoughts – change your life. Could it be that simple?

Take time to write out your own affirmations and bring them with you everywhere you go – place them in your purse, in your car, on your mirrors, in the fridge – get some Post-it notes today or a little notebook and always carry an affirmation with you!

WHAT ARE YOUR CURRENT AFFIRMATIONS?

'The moment
you change your
perception you can
change the chemistry
of your body'

– Dr Bruce Lipton

DARE OF THE DAY

Start each day with choosing **three** things to be grateful for – make it a daily habit! As you say your affirmations, focus on the positive emotions you feel around these people or events, the gratitude that you feel for these things happening.

TRY IT NOW

I am thankful for:

1. ....

....

....

2. ....

....

....

3. ....

....

....

DARE OF THE WEEK

This week, take time to examine your thoughts – to 'think' purposefully – and become more aware of them. Using a mantra or affirmation, try to keep your thoughts positive.

Here are seven affirmations: choose to say one a day for the next week and after you get the hang of them, try creating your own to suit your own life. Remember to keep them in this present moment and really believe them to be true.

1. All is well; everything is working out for my higher good.

2. I am in the right place at the right time doing the right thing.

3. I live my life with purpose and I make the best decisions for my life.

4. I am safe, secure and fully supported by the universe.

5. I am healthy and strong.

6. I am surrounded by loving relationships.

7. I love myself and I love my life.

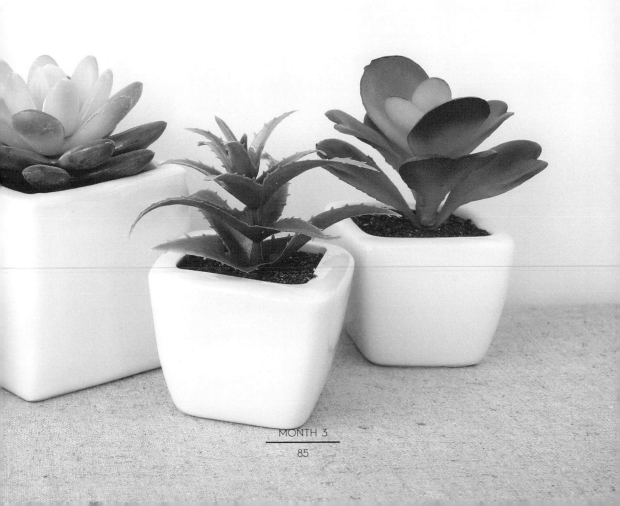

DARE OF THE MONTH

Practise trust: replace fearful thoughts about the future with a self-knowing. Use this **one-minute meditation** practice daily when you feel fear creeping into your thoughts.

ONE-MINUTE MEDITATION

Slowly inhale and slowly exhale, breathing deeply. As you breathe, say silently: *I breathe in trust and slowly exhale all fearful or negative thoughts.*

Repeat for about a minute, imagining all the time that trust is going right down into the bottom of your stomach and then to your toes, filling your body. Then imagine **exhaling all negativity**: expel it from your body and mind**.**

Continue to do this simple exercise until you feel the energy shift within you. Focus on all the positives and renew your trust in your higher power.

How did you feel after taking a minute to breathe and meditate?

MY PERSONAL EXPERIENCE WITH AFFIRMATIONS AND HOW I USED THEM IN MY DAILY LIFE:
extract from my journal

Today has been a day filled with art and craft! I have to say my bedroom looks a bit strange – I took a big, long chunk of Brooke's roll of paper, wrote my affirmations about my health goals on it and stuck it on the full-length mirror. I also put Post-it notes everywhere in the house and in my car with the affirmations written on them. I feel it will remind me to repeat them and it keeps me on track to write in my journal too.

I also have been making full use of my library card. I actually forgot how much I loved the library – it is an amazing place to spend an afternoon. So yesterday I got all my new books and I am reading about affirmations with Louise L. Hay and really exploring the whole concept of hypnosis. I love learning new things and it is broadening my horizons and outlook on life and healing. I also got a book about gratitude and how it affects your whole life, even in healing ways. The more we are happy for, the more we attract of that thing – isn't that such a powerful thought?

I am also really enjoying writing daily again and I am actually finding it is firing my creativity. I am thinking of doing a new course on healing and health and the power of the mind. The whole area is just really igniting my passion again for learning.

Could I deal more effectively with my pain using my mind? Mind over matter?

I have been doing more googling about hypnosis and some evidence suggests that the brain has the power to manipulate the body's physiology, so maybe I need to learn how to use my brain more effectively.

I believe in the power of the mind. I suppose that's why I can't get my head around the fact that I still have pain. Why can't I just use the power of positive thinking to overcome it? I think I will try. The future is looking and feeling very exciting. For now I am flexing my gratitude muscles.

Thank you, universe, for bringing these books into my world.

Thank you for all the love in my life.

Thank you for all the happiness and joy I share with David and Brooke.

Thank you for my health – I am feeling happier and healthier each day.

Thank you for all the little things that are bringing me happiness.

I am so grateful that I am learning new things each day about myself and about what I want in life.

Thank you, thank you, thank you, thank you, thank you, thank you for my life – it is a blessing.

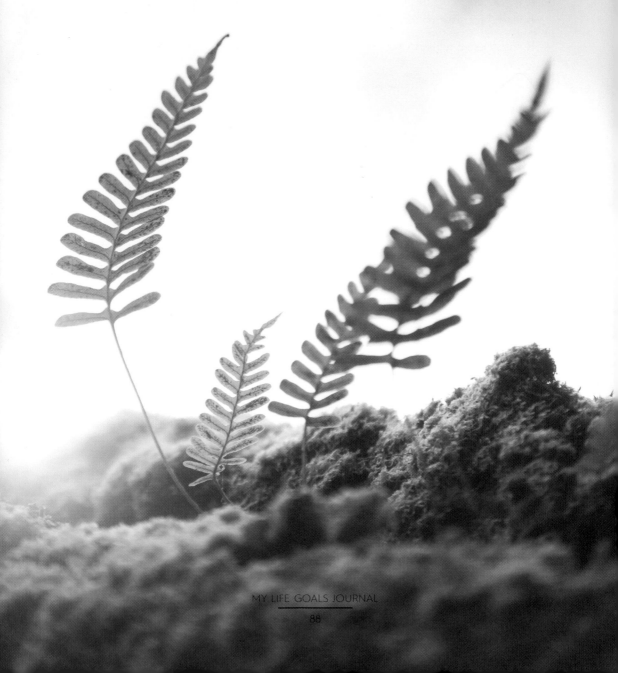

'It always seems
impossible until it's done.'

– Nelson Mandela

MONTHLY REVIEW

▸ This month's hypnosis relaxation will help you become consciously aware of how your thoughts can create your reality.

▸ Is it becoming a daily habit now to write in your journal? Or did you find you had some empty pages last month? Maybe ask yourself if you struggled with self-love. This month's theme brings our attention to our thoughts, so journal about how you feel day to day.

▸ Are you enjoying the daily hypnosis relaxation on my website? Have you noticed you are making time to listen to them every day?

▸ Remember, anything and everything is possible within your own personal journal.

PROMPTS

What are you thinking about right now?

If I could talk to my younger self the one thing I would say is:

If my body could talk to me it would say:

_____

_____

_____

_____

_____

_____

The words I live by are:

_____

_____

_____

_____

_____

_____

My Journal

_____

_____

_____

_____

_____

_____

_____

_____

_____

_____

_____

_____

'Just write every day of your life. Then see what happens.'

– Ray Bradbury

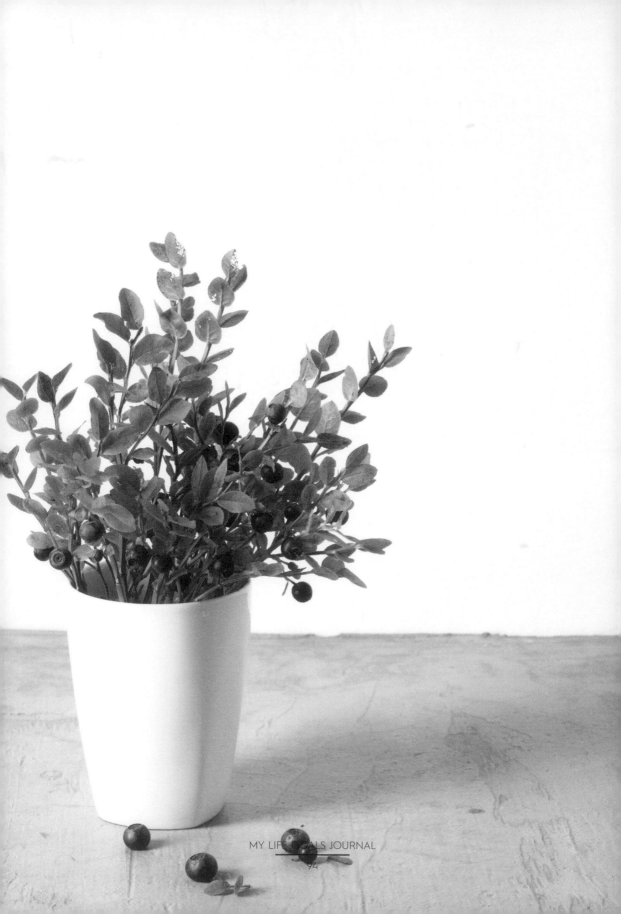

MONTH 4

Conscious eating and healthy living

'Let food be thy medicine
and medicine be thy food'

– Hippocrates

This month, consciously focus on everything that goes inside your body and, with it, your mind. After the first few months' exploring you should be feeling confident about who you are and creating the best version of yourself. By journaling and exploring your own creativity, new ideas and concepts will be percolating at a subconscious level – I am sure you are brimming with new possibilities.

Just as the seasons change, so do we, and as we embrace the new, we must be willing to let go of old habits and things that no longer serve us.

In many ways, through journaling and retraining our minds we are getting back to basics in all areas of our lives – it is the perfect time to focus on keeping things simple. As we simplify our lives we can eliminate habits that no longer serve our greater good.

Having come this far, now is the perfect time to declutter our lives – whether this means detoxing our body, our mind or our home – to create a more simple, streamlined existence.

Start with your diet

Try to **nourish** your body with simple, natural, fresh foods, and make an effort to drink as much water as you can every day. Declutter your diet by focusing on simple things. Sometimes it is easy to reach for a convenient snack, so avoid temptations and be prepared. Don't buy that packet of biscuits in your weekly shop; try some nuts or grains instead. Look for some sweet, juicy fruit instead of chocolate. By making small adjustments to your diet you can see real changes.

I decided to try to eat only vegetarian foods for one month and that simple act has changed my life, as I have never returned to eating meat. You can start in a smaller way by replacing white bread, rice and pasta with wholemeal or whole-wheat versions. Maybe make a conscious effort this month to switch tea and coffee for herbal alternatives or replace alcohol with sparkling water.

REMEMBER, IT IS SMALL HABITS
THAT BUILD OVER TIME THAT CAN
REALLY HAVE AN IMPACT ON YOUR
OVERALL WELLNESS.

———

CLEAN OUT YOUR FRIDGE
AND CUPBOARDS. YOU MIGHT
BE SURPRISED TO REALISE HOW
INCREDIBLY SATISFYING IT CAN
BE TO HAVE A GOOD CLEAR OUT!
ORGANISE EVERYTHING TIDILY USING
BOXES OR JARS; THROW AWAY
ANYTHING THAT IS OUT OF DATE.
DECLUTTER YOUR ENVIRONMENT
AND YOU WILL DECLUTTER YOUR
MIND, GIVING YOU A CLEARER
FOCUS.

———

TAKE TIME THIS WEEK TO
HONOUR THIS MONTH'S INTENTION
OF BECOMING MINDFUL OF THE
FOOD YOU PUT IN YOUR BODY.

'The food you eat can be either the safest and most powerful form of medicine or the slowest form of poison'

– Ann Wigmore

Make time for exercise

Do what is right for you and **listen to your body**. It could be as simple as walking or cycling to work. Maybe get off the bus a stop earlier to give yourself a little exercise in the morning. Perhaps a lunchtime jog or an exercise class after work is the answer. Make it your intention this month to be **fitter and healthier** in all your life choices – look for opportunities to get moving. Could you make a commitment to become active for thirty minutes three times a week? I felt I couldn't exercise because of my health issues but I had to recognise that I was using fear to avoid the issue. If, like me, you're stuck in an unhealthy routine, now is the time to get up, get out and **start moving**. This will benefit not only your body but also your mind – you might even get some enjoyment out of it too!

Rehydration

Keep a water bottle with some lemon and mint on your kitchen counter or beside your desk at work – make hydration your new habit!

Refuel

Think of your body like an engine: it cannot run on empty so make sure you provide your body with the essential nutrients it needs to stay healthy and well. Don't skip meals – always have a healthy go-to snack or protein shake ready for busy times. You could also ask for advice in your local health-food store about adding vitamins or supplements to your diet to maintain optimum health. Choose to put **wholesome, natural foods** into your body. Try to eat fresh, simple, healthy foods – it will keep your body and mind functioning at their optimal level.

Rejuvenate

Replace the old with the new – create new habits and reawaken your zest for life and living. To help build your new healthy habits, make your changes part of your routine and plan ahead. Maybe add a reward into reaching your wellness goals at the end of the week!

RECHARGE

Maybe it's time to kick-start a new health and exercise routine that will benefit your body and mind. Why not begin now?

My new healthy habit is ....

I will include it in my routine on .... at ....

I will reward myself with .... on completion of my weekly health goals.

USE THE LIST BELOW TO HELP YOU PLAN.

Make a list of the healthy food and exercise habits you would like to continue with on a regular basis:

1. ....

....

2. ....

....

3. ....

....

4. ....

....

5. ....

....

Healthy living

Detoxing our body can go hand in hand with a good home decluttering.

The **decluttering** journey doesn't need to be painful or difficult – it is a positive step towards a new you. Many people have come up with fun, creative ways to get started – you don't have to buy a book on it: you can google ideas or, more importantly, you can just get going. If you have clothes that you haven't worn for more than a year, do you need them?

Imagine you are clearing out some of the old to make way for the new and exciting. It might seem like a chore but all it takes is a little focused attention and a plan of action. You don't have to clear everything at once: decide to clear one area at a time in your home – one drawer, one cupboard or one closet.

Try to make an effort this month to declutter one thing each day – start with a shelf in your wardrobe and before you know it the whole area will be clear and tidy. Or start in your office with a book shelf or even your inbox on your computer. Trust me: this daily habit will have a huge effect on your overall wellness and peace of mind.

'Clutter is the physical manifestation of unmade decisions fueled by procrastination'

– Christina Scalise, *Organise Your Life and More*

ONE-YEAR RULE

If you haven't worn it/used it/looked at it in a year, get it out of your house!

BROKEN BEYOND REPAIR

It's broken, it's gone.

NOT EVEN YOURS

This is the worst type of clutter – you don't even own it! Give it back to the person who does.

'JUST IN CASE'

Think about the items you keep for this reason. Has any event come up where you actually needed them? If not, trust in the new you and get rid of them!

OUTDATED

There are items we are just done with but we haven't got around to getting rid of them. Now is that time.

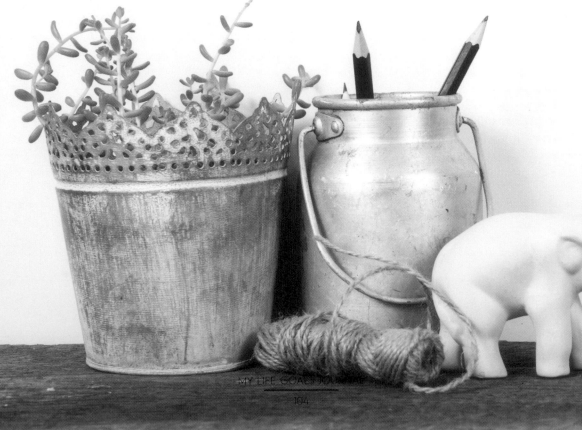

Your plan of attack – three simple steps

STEP 1

Before you start you need to get some boxes together – you will need lots of them. Label four boxes with the following:

* Rubbish
* Recycle
* Sell/donate
* Sort and file

Sort through the room and put purged items into the appropriate boxes – give as much as you can to a local charity if possible so someone else can benefit from your decluttering.

STEP 2

Organise the items you are keeping. Use containers, boxes or jars as necessary. If you are reorganising your wardrobe, make sure all the hangers are facing the same way and group clothes by style or colour. If you hang all your trousers together, think how much time you will save looking every morning.

STEP 3

Disposal! Moving things from one room to another isn't really decluttering. You have to follow through. Don't leave all the boxes at the bottom of the stairs: make time to plan a trip to ensure they leave your house!

'Out of clutter, find simplicity'

– Albert Einstein

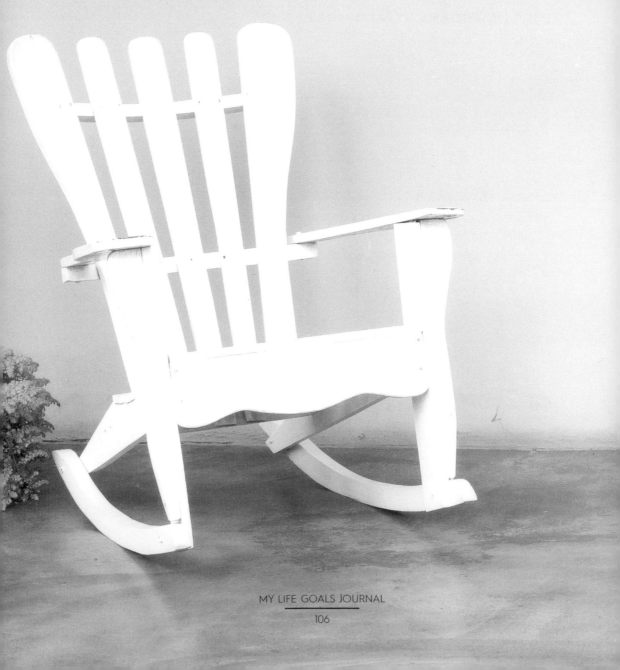

DARE OF THE DAY

Start today with a glass of water with lemon and, just for today, try to drink eight glasses of water.

DARE OF THE WEEK

This week, take time to 'think' purposefully about the food you eat. Plan your meals for the week and maybe make food in batches and freeze some.

FOOD I WOULD LIKE TO EAT THIS WEEK:

FOOD I WOULD LIKE TO AVOID THIS WEEK:

7-DAY MEAL PLAN

DAY	BREAKFAST	LUNCH	DINNER
MON			
TUES			
WED			
THURS			
FRI			
SAT			
SUN			

GROCERY LIST

FRUIT	VEGGIES	PROTEIN	GRAINS	OTHER

DARE OF THE MONTH

Make it your intention to exercise: sign up to a new gym or swimming class or walking club **today**. For this month, track your activity in an exercise journal. Make a decluttering plan for your home and track your success as you work through the list.

DECLUTTERING LIST:

MY HEALTHY NEW DIET:
extract from my journal

It seems a bit strange starting a diet mid-year, but that's what I am doing. For this month I am becoming a vegan. I have been looking up courses and on one of my recent date days to the beach I stopped off at a shop I love – to my surprise they are running a four-week vegan cookery course. I went straight online and signed myself up.

That's the third course I have committed to in recent days and I'm feeling a mixture of fear and exaltation about it. I love the idea of vegetarianism but hadn't considered the idea of becoming a vegan. I actually think it is the universe sending me signs, which sounds weird, but it seems everything I am reading or researching is pointing me in that direction. I have just picked up a book from the library called The China Study by T. Colin Campbell, who is Jacob Gould Schurman Professor Emeritus at Cornell University. If I am honest, it looks very serious and very scientific but actually it explores the relationship between a rich animal-based diet and illness and disease in the body. I've only flicked through it in recent days, and I was thinking that eliminating all dairy as well as meat would be impossible, so I didn't really consider it until today. Then suddenly I stumble upon the vegan course! Coincidentally, the course I have booked later in the year with Doreen Virtue will also touch on becoming a vegan. It is like I am being divinely guided.

So my plan for tomorrow is to declutter my cupboards and fridge in preparation for the course on Wednesday. I actually cannot remember the last time I did that, and I am sure there is so much stuff that is out of date in there.

I had a quick look before I came to bed and it really inspired me to do it properly tomorrow. The whole idea of things reaching their expiry date and still being in the cupboard is actually a good reflection of where I am at the moment in life. I am really starting to look at everything and question whether it is useful and if I really need it in my life – and it isn't just food.

I find myself looking at relationships and even at work. Do I get value from doing this or am I just bored and really not getting any nutrition mentally from doing it? Could I be doing something else or eating something else that would fill me with more goodness? It sounds silly but actually thinking about decluttering tomorrow *has made me think about other areas of my life and even just writing now in my journal is making me think more. I think I might do an entire life audit and streamline my world. Isn't it amazing how just writing stuff out and committing that stream of consciousness to paper can excavate gold nuggets of information and self-reflection?*

I am becoming so much more fluid and open in my daily journal writing and I really am allowing the words to flow from a place of honesty. Writing freely without judgement has brought so many revelations into my world.

I must remember to adopt that same non-judgemental attitude to my new vegan diet that I am going to embrace. I feel it is an exciting opportunity to detox and also get healthy. I shall write about my experience and hopefully in time I will be recording the health benefits.

'Be the change that you wish
to see in the world'

– Mahatma Gandhi

MONTHLY REVIEW

- This hypnosis relaxation will help you make healthier food and lifestyle choices.

- Have you lots of ideas about areas in your life that you might like to declutter? Remember this month's theme is all about being as healthy as you can in your mind and body.

- If you are having trouble setting new healthy goals, the daily hypnosis relaxation will help you focus.

- Be honest about your own feelings in the journal pages and maybe ask yourself how consciously you are eating and how healthy your lifestyle is.

PROMPTS

Ask yourself how consciously you are eating:

I feel most energised when:

When did you feel at your healthiest and why?

Begin a food journal to help you track the food you eat:

My Journal

'Writing is medicine. It is an
appropriate antidote to injury. It is
an appropriate companion for any
difficult change.'
— Julia Cameron

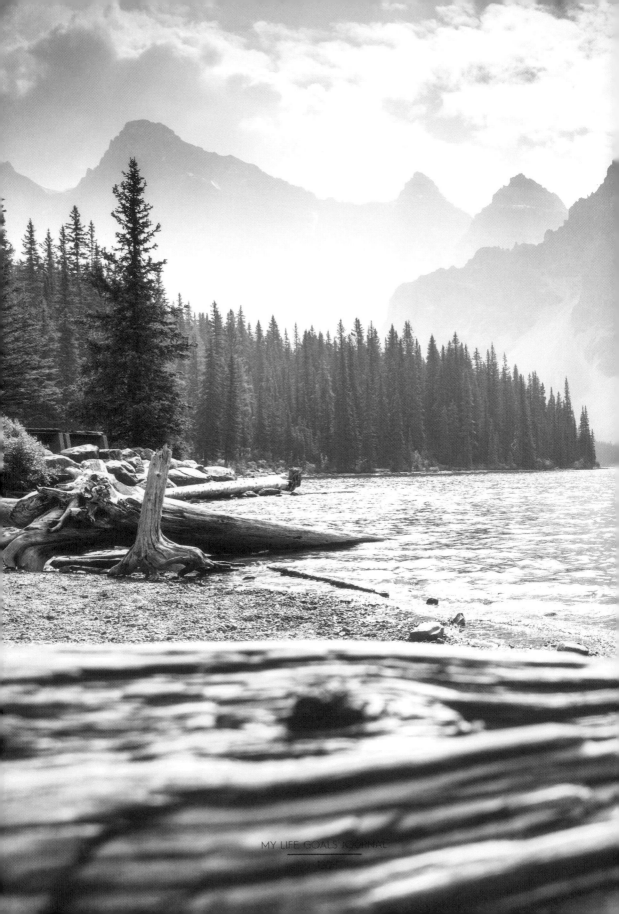

MONTH 5

Self-talk

'None but ourselves can free our minds'

—Bob Marley

The Science of Self-Talk

The **power of our thoughts** was the subject of debate and discussion even in biblical times. This is highlighted in a verse in the Bible from the Book of Proverbs, 23:7 – **'As a man thinketh in his heart, so is he.'**

This is perhaps the most basic statement of how I believe our minds work: our minds will believe everything we tell them, so this month make a conscious effort to **feed your mind positive ideas** of love and joy and visions of abundance.

I couldn't believe how much negative self-talk I was using around my health and my lifestyle, and it was going on all day on a subconscious level. To my surprise, my negative self-talk accounted for as much as 80 per cent of my daily chitchat to myself. Stopping this, focusing on the positive through affirmations and controlling my negative energy has had a huge effect on my psyche and my health.

Try to be aware that you may be repeating negative thoughts that become 'affirmations' without thinking. For example, I believed and often unconsciously repeated the affirmations, both in my mind and when speaking to people, that 'I am losing power in my arm' or 'I am just not able'. I said these so often that, unknowingly, I was making my brain believe they were true.

I challenge you to pay attention to your self-talk for the next day and see what your self-talk is telling you. What percentage of it is positive, do you think? What percentage of it is negative?

Think about what you are thinking right now. What do those thoughts say about you? About your life? And how well do they really match your plans for your life and how you imagine yourself in the future?

Our inner dialogue tells a story: we can decide right now if that will be positive or negative. There are a few ways you can develop better **self-talk**, the first step, is to acknowledge your internal conversations. So simply start by actively listening to what you're saying to yourself each day, notice if it is positive or negative and become aware if it is having an impact on how you feel, physically and mentally.

Positive self-talk is the stuff that makes you feel good about yourself and the things that are going on in your life. It is like having an optimistic voice in your head that looks on the bright side, gives you compliments and truly believes in you!

Negative self-talk is the stuff that makes you feel pretty bad about yourself and the things that are going on in your life. This is like having a constant negative voice judging you, telling you that you're not good enough and making you feel miserable.

Being positive all the time isn't achievable – and probably isn't helpful – but self-talk is more than a confidence booster. From a neuroscientific perspective, it is a form of internal remodelling.

WHAT IS YOUR SELF TALK RIGHT NOW?

'A journey of a thousand miles begins with a single step
If you correct your mind the rest will fall into place'

– Lao Tzu

How can you make your self-talk work for you?

We don't always consciously take note of what we're saying to ourselves, but there are a few things you can do to help change the direction of your self-talk.

Ask yourself now, 'What limiting beliefs are holding me back?' Answering that question is key to breaking through to the life you really want. A great test is to make a 'can't' list: a list of what you 'know' you can't do and why.

TRY THIS EXERCISE

Complete the following sentence for everything that comes to mind:

I **can't** .... **because** ....

....

....

....

....

....

....

....

Pay attention to what comes after the word 'because'. That's your own inner voice telling you that there is a reason this is impossible. That inner voice is what keeps you from being open to possibility.

I believed I **couldn't** live a pain-free life **because** my doctors told me my pain wasn't going away.

I believed that I **couldn't** write a book **because** this seemed like something other people did, not someone like me. I didn't think I was smart enough or that my English was up to the standard required for a published book.

Often times we hold onto statements that are imprinted onto our subconscious mind since childhood about our abilities and this can hold us back in our adult life. For me, I was told by someone as a child that I wasn't a good singer and I believed this to be true.

I later made it my intention to improve on my singing by joining a choir.

Many things we might believe to be impossible can become possible if we challenge our internal negative dialogue about them.

DARE OF THE DAY

Set aside five minutes to write out all the positive things about yourself: what you can do really well, everything you like about yourself physically, mentally and even spiritually – think about all your skills and achievements as far back as childhood.

Allow yourself to write non-stop for the **full five minutes** – do not think about spelling or censoring what you jot down: just keep your pen writing and don't lift it from the page until the five minutes are up – set an alarm if you need to.

'If you can dream it,
you can do it'

– Walt Disney

DARE OF THE WEEK

Feed your mind. Trust that you are starting to consciously form new neural pathways with your positive thoughts. If you find it hard to say positive things to yourself, this week write down some examples and get into the habit of saying them.

I CAN ACHIEVE MY GOALS THIS WEEK OF:

1. ....

2. ....

3. ....

4. ....

5. ....

I BELIEVE IN MYSELF AND I KNOW I CAN:

1. ....

2. ....

3. ....

4. ....

5. ....

I AM FEELING FANTASTIC AND I AM CAPABLE OF GREAT THINGS LIKE:

1. ....

2. ....

3. ....

4. ....

5. ....

Replace your inner self-critical voice with self-love and acceptance. The more you work on improving your self-talk the better you will get. It is like starting anything new: it won't be easy at first, but it will get better with time.

Note to self
– You are unique and brilliant

Note to self
– Learn from your past and don't let it define your future

Note to self
– I am enough

Note to self
– I am in the process of positive change in my life

DARE OF THE MONTH

Positively reframe any observations made by your inner critic. Once you start to notice your inner voice at work you will quickly spot when it begins to be negative. Immediately force yourself to speak more positively – treat yourself like you would a young child or your best friend and speak with love. While engaging in this supportive self-talk, you might find it helpful to have some positive notes to yourself to keep with you. This month, write loving, encouraging notes on pieces of paper and bring them with you. I have included some here and you can make up your own personal ones.

WRITE YOUR OWN NOTE

'Kind words can be short and easy to speak, but their echoes are truly endless'

– Mother Teresa

SOME TIPS FOR POSITIVE SELF-TALK

⁕ Make a conscious effort to **think positive**. Statements like 'I know I can do it', 'I am filled with positive energy right now' or 'I know I can achieve anything I put my mind to' can help your brain pick up the positive cues.

⁕ Start to **question your self-talk**. Ask things like: 'What would I say if a friend were in a similar situation?' 'Is there a more positive way of looking at this?' 'Can I do anything to change what I'm feeling bad about?'

⁕ **Change your self-talk**. Consciously change the negative self-talk into positive self-talk. When you notice negative self-talk, say to yourself, 'No. Stop.' Then replace the negative thought with a positive one. For example, if you think, 'I'll never be able to do this,' ask yourself, **'Is there anything I can do that will help me be able to do this?'** Believe in yourself and trust that everything is working out for your good.

⁕ Use **balanced thinking**. It can be a tough battle at the beginning, but when you make it a habit to listen to that inner voice, you can change your life in miraculous ways. Remember, your subconscious mind will always believe everything you tell it.

⁕ **Motivational self-talk** means using encouraging phrases like: 'Come on!' 'Let's go!' 'You can do this!' 'You will do your walk today.' Use it to help you achieve what you want.

⁕ **Instructional self-talk** is helpful when practising a task like journaling. You instruct yourself until it becomes automatic. For example, you might tell yourself that you will aim to write one page before lunchtime, or that you know and believe that the daily affirmations will be of benefit if you stick with them. Remind yourself to listen to one of the hypnosis downloads on my website. Doing all of these things is reprogramming your mind to think positively.

After several weeks you will eventually form the blueprint for changing how you relate to yourself long-term and this powerful act of reframing your self-talk will change your life.

MY NOTE WRITTEN TO MYSELF:
extract from my journal

I am feeling a little alone. All this stuff I am doing is internal, and it's very much a solitary journey, one I have been taking by myself, changing my perceptions and inner dialogue. It is really beneficial and I can see changes but sometimes I am a little impatient. I want things to move quicker.

I know it is hard to change your life overnight, but maybe because I am doing all this work and it isn't immediately obvious, I am doubting myself and asking myself if it is really making any difference.

I have to keep myself grounded and remind myself that **yes** it is working and I am making huge changes in my life and that requires patience. Because I have been honest about my feelings of isolation and loneliness, I want to try to deal with them and remind myself I am doing a good job. I've decided I am going to write a message to myself and text it to my own number so I can remember it when I am out and about and I have moments of doubt. This is the message I will send: 'Andrea, you are enough.' I took my inspiration from Maya Angelou's quote 'You alone are enough. You have nothing to prove to anybody.'

My mind can be my biggest critic and, without actually even realising, I suddenly hear my inner voice berating this journey I am on and saying things like, 'this will never work', 'you're wasting your time', 'you won't be able to complete that course', 'you can't achieve that goal'. It might only be a fleeting thought but I have noticed that the thought can begin a chain reaction of negative feelings and suddenly I am feeling lonely like I was earlier. Instead of feeling alone I need to be my own best friend and talk more kindly to myself.

Dear Andrea,
I wanted to write this note to say I am so proud of you – you are doing an amazing job looking after your health and wellness and everything you are doing is enough.
Andrea, don't feel you always have to be strong. It is OK to feel lonely or scared; it is OK to allow tears to flow when they need to.
You are taking charge of your own life and that takes courage. I love your

courage – to try something new, to follow your heart, to give generously, to acknowledge you need help sometimes and to know it is OK to cry.

Andrea, you took back control and now no one is in charge of your happiness except you! And you are choosing to be happy and healthy.

Thank you for trusting your heart over your head. Even when it meant taking time off work to make your wellness a priority, you took a risk, embraced the unknown and allowed new things to manifest in your life – that takes guts and I love you for that.

Andrea, you are brave enough to gracefully let go of things that no longer serve you. Even if it means saying no to work and yes to yourself, thank you for putting yourself first and becoming the best version of yourself.

Thank you for trusting in yourself and achieving whatever you put your mind to: you are healthier than ever and still on track to achieve your medication and health goals – well done, you.

Andrea, you are never alone: do not feel lonely. Instead know there is always something brilliant going on in your mind – a mixture of intentions, dreams, hopes and ideas that you are creating and manifesting every moment: focus on those. Your mind is a sacred place where everything is possible: stay on track and trust you are doing everything right. Even when you doubt yourself on this journey, look back to the beginning and congratulate yourself on how far you have already come.

'What you think you become, what you feel you attract, what you imagine you create.'

Lots of love,
Andrea x

'Turn your wounds into wisdom. You don't become what you want, you become what you believe'

– Oprah

MONTHLY REVIEW

‣ This month's hypnosis relaxation will help you become more mindful of your inner dialogue and teach you to engage in positive self-talk.

‣ As we approach the halfway point in this journal, are you enjoying filling the pages with your own personal entries? This month's theme of self-talk should help you become more self-aware, and this might alter your writing style.

‣ Have you noticed the daily hypnosis relaxations on my website are getting a little longer? Don't forget you can mix and match the themes and use them as you need them.

‣ The power of the pen is very evident in journaling so keep going and make it your intention to read over some old entries too.

PROMPTS

Reframe any of your old thoughts about yourself to make them more positive:

If you could change one thing about your present life what would it be?

What is the dominant emotion in your life right now?

My Journal

'The act of writing is the act of
discovering what you believe.'
              – David Hare

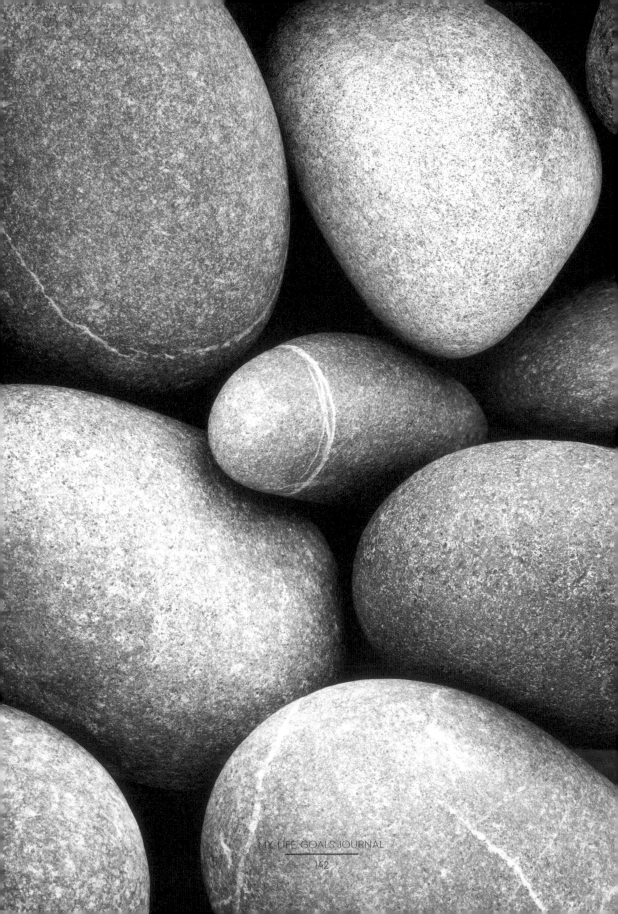

MONTH 6

Manifestation and abundance

'Our intention creates
our reality'

– Wayne Dyer

This month make it your intention to look for the riches in your life. The first wealth is health – a healthy mind, body and soul make for a richer you.

By focusing on all the good things you already have you will attract more abundance into your life – this is known as the **law of attraction**. Just imagine for a moment that you can create your reality, that you can get whatever you want, that you can manifest anything. How wonderful would your life be? It's a powerful thought, isn't it?

Just for a moment, imagine we are responsible in some way for creating the reality around us.

Sometimes it seems impossible to believe such a thing, but if you look at your life, in many ways the choices and decisions you have made in the past have informed where you are now.

If you want to manifest abundance in all areas of your life then start now by embracing new intentions about your reality. Stop focusing on anything you lack; instead concentrate your mind on the wealth of positives in your world.

Every day is a chance to start a new page in your life or a new chapter in your life's purpose: make today's entry exciting and great; dare to manifest abundance in all areas of your life.

TODAY I WOULD LIKE TO MANIFEST:

TRY THIS EXERCISE TO HELP YOU FOCUS

My thoughts that have become my reality ...

1. ....

2. ....

3. ....

4. ....

5. ....

6. ....

7. ....

8. ....

This has worked for me. In the spirit of New Year challenges, I wrote down a list of things and situations I wanted to manifest. I made it my intention to attract what my mind was thinking into my life. I became very aware of the things I wanted to manifest, and that self-awareness was the catalyst for change. I have truly transformed and my life has too. I am now an **empowered** person who is living a happier and healthier life than ever before. Here is my list of my thoughts that have become my reality.

1. Health

I wanted to manifest an abundance of health. I suffer from constant pain, but up to 2014 I hadn't really looked at how many other areas in my life were suffering as a result of this. I just tried to put my best face forward day to day, while behind the smiles I was just existing and getting through the days. In 2014 I realised I really wanted to start to live a fulfilled life of joy and abundance. So I began to seek more balance in every area of my life.

2. Work

I knew believing I could manifest extraordinary change was central to my success. I took time out to monitor if I was living purposefully, reviewing what I had achieved on my journey and the things I still had to focus on. This really worked for me and I believe it can work for you too. If I can make big changes in my life, I promise you, so can you. For me, I began to write my story, which formed my book. I began to think about the content and worked every day to make my goal of a finished manuscript become a reality.

3. Weight

I had the thought and intention of losing weight and feeling great so I allowed my mind to create and visualise the perfect, healthy, fit version of myself. In fact I searched for old pictures of me at my perfect body size and imagined myself being that healthy size again. This became my motivation to make healthy decisions about my diet and it encouraged me to include a little exercise in my day-to-day life. Over time I did achieve the weight I wanted although it did take a commitment to my vision.

4. Leisure

I also decided I wanted to enjoy more downtime and this meant I needed to plan and prioritise family holiday time. I sat down with my husband and looked at the year ahead and started to map out when we would take holidays. In the past we often left it until the last minute, when air fares were at a premium, and sometimes we missed out on holidays because of cost. So we set a budget at the start of the year, planned accordingly and actually got some great deals – but it took time, dedication and forward planning. I have lots of lovely photos to remind me of those happy holidays which I intended to manifest.

5. Finances

I decided to try to stick to a budget so I could save money for my holidays, which I wanted to enjoy. Again, this is all part of planning ahead and looking at how you can do things to make savings every day. For me, I stopped buying a coffee every day and brought one in my own travel mug. Over time, little changes like bringing your own lunch into work or getting the bus instead of a taxi will all begin to accumulate.

Make it your **intention** to manifest the things you want to attract: this month expect plenty of great opportunities to flow easily to you.

Look back at some of the goals you set at the start of the year. Are you heading towards them or do you need to take stock and perhaps change direction a little? I always believe that if I can think it, I can do it – make that work for you.

'If my mind can conceive it,
and my heart can believe it –
then I can achieve it'

– Muhammad Ali

RE-EVALUATE THE NEXT 6 MONTHS

Make a list of areas you want to **refocus** on. Maybe you're struggling day to day to manage your time? Now could be a good opportunity to re-examine your life and see where you need to turn your attention to.

You can read my examples in my journal entry at the end of this month.

1.
2.
3.
4.
5.
6.

Review your priorities. It might be that you are spending all your time on a demanding work schedule or your responsibilities at home – could you create more balance in certain areas of your life?

In my case, I needed to accept I wasn't making my health a priority and I need to make time for my daily walk.

1.
2.
3.
4.
5.
6.

Reset, **rethink** and **pre-plan** to tackle these issues. If you notice you aren't balanced in a certain area, you need to make changes. How can you implement your new goals?

In order to make time for my daily walk, I needed to set my alarm earlier so I could get it done before my busy day started.

1. ....

2. ....

3. ....

4. ....

5. ....

6. ....

Revise and **rearrange** your goals. What will you tackle first?

Look back over the goals that you have set and see if you have achieved any. Once they're crossed off the list, you can set new ones. Or maybe a goal has taken more time than expected. Analyse why and take further steps to making your goal a reality.

When my health was more in balance, I could set new goals in other areas of my life – you can do this too.

1. ....

2. ....

3. ....

4. ....

5. ....

6. ....

DARE OF THE DAY

Take time to become mindful of the positive things that you already have brought into life: like your relationships, friendships and your successes.

Find a space where you won't be disturbed. Take a few minutes to clear your mind and centre yourself. We'll begin with three deep, long breaths.

1. Take a deep breath in, count to three then breathe out slowly.
2. Do this again, and this time when you breathe in think of the word **abundance** and when you breathe out think of all the **riches** in your life.
3. Finally, on your third breath, breathe in **manifestation** and think of what you want to attract into your life and then breathe out **confidence** that this will become your reality.

Now with a clear vision of what you want, write your wish for the day and trust you can manifest it:

Take a deep breath in.

I wish to attract ....

....

....

....

As you breathe out, imagine the feelings you will have when your wish becomes a reality.

I will feel ....

....

....

....

When you truly feel and visualise what you wish to manifest, you are sending out energy to the universe to bring that intention back to you by using the secret law of attraction. I believe that like attracts like – it is a magnetic force, a law of nature, not a miracle!

DARE OF THE WEEK

This week, explore the ritual of sending an 'order' for what you want to manifest into the universe: it is your wish list of abundance!

MANIFESTATION EXERCISE

Step one – define and write down what you want to manifest.
Step two – have a strong desire for that outcome to happen.
Step three – send it out into the universe! There are a few ways to send your wish out into the cosmos: put the piece of paper into the ocean or bury it in the soil – or simply trust that your order has been heard.
Allow the universe to manifest your outcome without worrying about how it's to be achieved.

SAY GOODBYE TO NEGATIVE ENERGY

To remove any negative, fear-based thoughts attached to creating your wish list, the powerful ritual of **burning** to transmute negative energy can be effective. It might seem a little bit silly but the act can be very powerful and symbolic.

Write a list of your **fears** or anything you feel is holding you back. Set the list alight – simply and carefully watch your negative fear-based emotions to go up in smoke and allow the energy to be **released** and **removed** from you.

Visualisation is a very efficient technique that can be used alongside this process. For example, simply **visualise** that you are filling the room, or your aura if you are outside, with clear white light that is removing all negative energies as the smoke from the burning list is flushed out into the universe.

You can also use essential oils of **sage** or a sage stick. The aroma of sage increases the oxygen supply to the brain, producing a relaxation of muscle tension. The act of burning sacred herbs to transmute negative energy can also be used to help the process of manifestation and attracting great abundance.

'If something you want is slow to come to you, it can only be for one reason: You are spending more time focused upon its absence than you are about its presence'

– Abraham-Hicks

DARE OF THE MONTH

For many people manifestation is about success and abundance can be about prosperity, so begin to live as though you have already attracted what you wanted.

- **For prosperity** – show your money how much you love it by creating a safe environment for it to feel valued in your purse or wallet. Make sure you arrange your banknotes in order and keep them unfolded. Throw away any old receipts or expired cards – clear the dead energy. This process gives the universe a very clear message that you have created space for more abundance to be drawn to you effortlessly.

- **For success** – if you want a new job or change in career, update your CV this month and make it your intention to network and let people in your business know you are looking to move. Arrange a meeting with a recruitment consultant or send your CV out to attract the perfect job.

- **For love** – trust that today could be the day you meet your lifelong partner, so make an effort to look as you would if you were going on a date. Maybe join a dating site or make it your intention to go out and join a new social group – get out and mix socially this month. Trust and believe that the perfect person is going to come into your life – make a list of all the qualities you want to attract in a perfect mate and let the universe know that this is your ideal partner.

BEGINNING TO SEE THE BENEFITS OF
THE LIFE I WAS MANIFESTING:
extract from my journal

While I am off work, focusing fully on my wellness, I have been doing lots of research on the power of the mind. I have read about athletes who claim it helps them perform better when they play the game in their minds before ever setting foot on the field or court. Playing the race, game or sport over in their mind as a mental exercise enables them to better focus on the day.

I'm wondering if there might be more concrete changes happening inside the body? I want to explore the whole concept of visualisation, relaxation and meditation alongside my hypnosis. I am excited about the possibilities.

Hand in hand with my own hypnosis sessions, I am actually now considering studying clinical hypnosis. I know it is a little shocking to even write it, but I want to manifest it somehow. The results I am getting with my own hypnosis sessions are amazing; I couldn't have predicted six months ago that I would be actually here and believing so much in the power of my own mind to change my life. Even writing that down is making me so excited for the next six months – what new opportunities and changes are around the corner?

My own focus has shifted a little because I am seeing such great changes in my own wellness and pain management.

I am beginning to open myself up to new things I would not have even thought about before, like studying clinical hypnosis.

I now need to rethink my goals and truly focus on making my intention of studying hypnosis a reality.

I will need to research training options in Ireland and draw up a plan of action to make it happen. I am actually so excited about it. I somehow **know** deep inside I will do this. I am making it my intention to achieve this goal somehow.

Over the next six months I want to refocus on:

1. Studying clinical hypnosis
2. Exploring more alternative healing modalities and training options
3. Going to mass every morning and expanding and getting in touch with my spirituality

I want to review and take time to prioritise:

1. Learning more about hypnosis study options and finding a mentor
2. My new hobbies/passions and allowing these new passions to blossom by making time to learn more or train more
3. Dedicating time each week to my spirituality and learning more about it

I need to:

1. Try to find a course to start in September in clinical hypnosis
2. Take a course on reiki training
3. Join a new group in the church

'In any given moment we have two options: to step forward into growth or to step back into safety'

– Abraham Maslow

MONTHLY REVIEW

▸ This month's hypnosis relaxation will help attract wonderful new opportunities to create the life you truly want to live.

▸ Are you seeing the positive benefits of actively using your journal? It is important to try to keep the momentum going, even if you only write a few words or just use pictures to illustrate your journey.

▸ Are you enjoying the hypnosis relaxations? The theme this month is abundance. Let me know if you have been manifesting change – share your experiences on my website.

▸ Is journaling now just a daily habit for you? Or do you still need to be prompted?

PROMPTS

What areas of your life are abundant and in what areas do you see lack?

What thing could you do every day that would make you fulfilled?

If you could manifest change in your life what would that be?

_____

_____

_____

_____

_____

_____

_____

_____

_____

_____

_____

_____

_____

_____

_____

My Journal

'Don't think it, ink it.'
  – Mark Victor Hansen

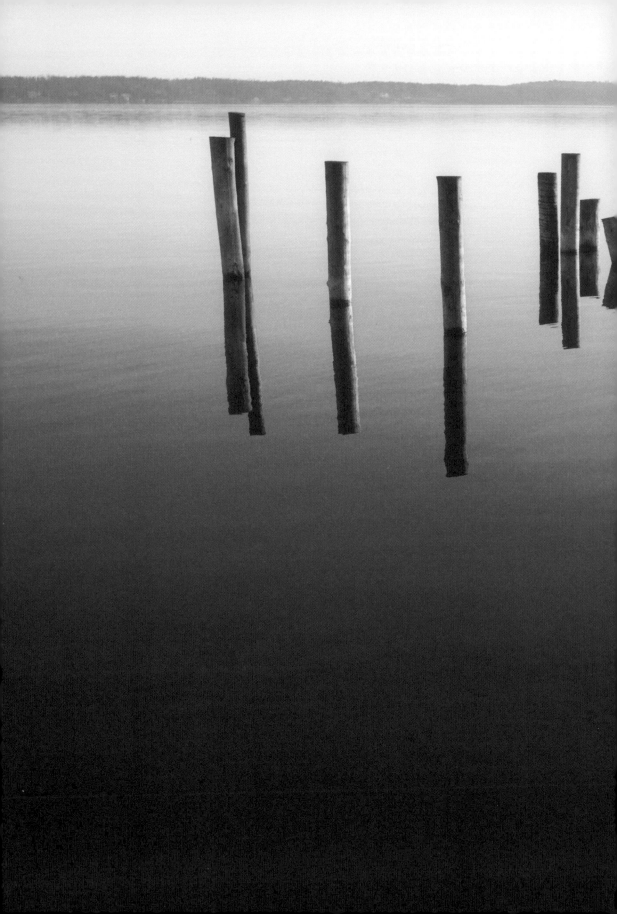

MONTH 7

Mindfulness
and nature

'Life is not measured by the number of breaths we take but by the moments that take our breath away'

– Maya Angelou

Go into this month with the attitude of peace in your mind, body and soul. You have learned how to treat yourself like your own best friend and live in your own sacred space of peace. Now look beyond yourself to the abundance and beauty in the **natural world** around you. Open your eyes, go outside, bathe in the sunshine, taste the rain, feel the wind, touch the sand and walk barefoot on the grass – enjoy all that nature has to offer.

Think about the little things in life that bring you **joy** and **happiness**. I love my morning walk with my dog Dash – I enjoy walking in all weathers and watching the seasons change from week to week. As a family we enjoy walking on the beach and collecting stones and shells – these simple pleasures bring me immense joy and inner calmness and I treasure those moments.

You do not know what this month will bring, but you can make it your **intention** to be mindful of your choices. We cannot live in the future or constantly keep reliving the past so we need to embrace the here and now and choose to be happy in this moment and reach for thoughts that will bring us to a happy space, right now.

Being mindful is about living in the moment and being aware of your thoughts. The whole notion of **mindfulness** has become very popular in recent years, but it can be simply defined as being completely in the here and now.

> Mindfulness is about focusing in this moment on how you feel, being with your thoughts as they are and being more conscious of life as it happens.

How often has a day gone by without your mind really savouring any special moments? All too often we eat our meals without even tasting the food; we go through our days on autopilot. Staying present is a battle, particularly in the throes of juggling busy, stressful lives and constant racing thoughts about the future.

It is not possible to live in the moment all the time but with a little practice it can happen more often than you imagine. Have you ever just lost yourself in a task? You were concentrating fully, you thought of nothing else and the world disappeared. This is the level of concentration we are trying to achieve, by focusing ourselves on how we feel, on what is going on around us.

Mindfulness can help us all become **calmer**, more **peaceful** and **focused** on the positives in our lives. By simply taking things day by day, hour by hour, minute by minute and moment by moment, you are choosing to stay centred in the here and now. Marrying this with positive thinking can make a huge difference to your mind, body and spirit.

You can bring the art of mindfulness into all areas of your life by taking some time to simply be.

HOW DOES IT FEEL TO TAKE A MINDFUL MOMENT?

- Take a few moments to concentrate on your **breathing** — notice the rise and fall of your belly and feel the air coming in and out of your lungs

- Tune into your **senses** — using all your senses concentrate on the touch, taste, sight, smell or texture all around you

- Notice your thoughts — just **accept** them and allow them to meander without trying to control or change them

- When your mind wanders, bring yourself back to your centre with your breathing — once again try to go back to the **present** moment

'When you do something beautiful and nobody noticed, don't be sad. For the sun every morning is a beautiful spectacle and yet most of the audience still sleeps'

– John Lennon

DARE OF THE DAY

Try to sit and be still in nature today for a few minutes. Find a safe place to focus your attention on your breath. Start **breathing** in and out slowly, without effort – allow each breath to come and go with ease. Let go of thoughts about things you have to do or commitments you need to attend to later in the day. Just sit in silence and be still in nature.

Breathe in this day, inhale its greatness, savour the experiences of today, as it will only last twenty-four hours and then be gone forever.

DARE OF THE WEEK

I have always used **walking** as a way to centre my thoughts, to really become mindful and to appreciate my life and all around me. Breathing and mindful walking go hand in hand. This week, take some time to yourself for a walk outside and try to breathe in a similar rhythm to your walking; make sure your shoulders and body posture are relaxed and you are really concentrating on each breath and each step you take.

Remember, it is easy to let your mind wander off, but when you notice you are thinking about something in the past or the future **centre yourself** with your breathing and bring yourself back to the here and now. Be aware of all your senses and keep your attention on everything around you and seeing yourself in that space.

Try to be aware of the beauty and wonder in all of creation. Try to walk on the grass or sand barefoot, really rejoice in the sounds and sights of nature and open your eyes to the magnificence in all living things.

DARE OF THE MONTH

Whatever the weather, get outdoors. Take an early morning walk or go out at dusk. Choose a lovely location where you can hear the breeze in the trees or waves lapping on the shore. Find solitude and sit peacefully meditating and being in the moment. Remember to breathe in and out slowly for a few minutes. Deep breaths are love notes to our bodies and you will feel grounded and peaceful with every breath. Enjoy the beauty around you.

Tip: If you can bring a camera or phone, take a photograph of where you are to remind you of each of the things that tickled your senses. You can include these photos into your journal too.

'In today's rush, we all think too much – seek too much – want too much – and forget about the joy of just being'

– Eckhart Tolle

Allow your body to receive all the glorious gifts that surround us in each moment by tuning into your senses.

1. **Taste** – Savour each bite and focus on the taste of everything you eat. Being mindful when you are eating is so important and will help you to slow down and aid your digestion.

2. **Sight** – So many of us walk with our heads down, buried in electronic gadgets, without even realising we are missing the beauty all around us. Look up to the horizon: start to notice how the seasons change the landscape around you.

3. **Sound** – Pay attention to everything you hear; close your eyes and allow yourself to absorb all of the sounds around you.

4. **Touch** – Notice different surfaces; try to practise becoming aware of everything that is touching your body, from the warmth of the sun on your face to the texture of the sand beneath your bare feet. Feel the fabric of your clothes; become aware of the moment.

5. **Smell** – Appreciate the smells around you. Take time to ground yourself in nature and become mindful of these sensual, earthy experiences. Enjoy the wonder and true miracle of nature and being in the present moment.

FINDING INSPIRATION IN NATURE:
extract from my journal

I decided to write my journal outside today and came here – to Powerscourt Gardens – to look for some solitude in nature. I arrived at the Japanese gardens asking for guidance and heaven's help from the angels. I am aware I am taking new, unexpected paths in my life at the moment and sometimes I can feel a little bit overwhelmed and scared of the changes that I am trying to implement.

Something amazing has happened as I walked around the gardens. I had an overwhelming realisation about life – just like the garden paths here that intertwine and mix together, there is no wrong way to go through life, and each path we take will eventually bring us to the same place in the end: our destiny.

Each time when I believed I had found the most beautiful walkway, I was totally taken by surprise when I saw the incredible beauty of nature waiting for me around the corner. I feel a sense of relief now, as I feel the lesson I am here to learn is that life is for living one day at a time. I need to simply take time to enjoy the beauty around me; I need to stop worrying about how to get to the end of the paths, to a destination or a place in my journey in life.

Each time we take new paths in our life new beauty and new options are revealed and in the end we will get to where we are meant to go.

Isn't it funny that as I walk here in this wonderful place I also realise my life is lacking beauty and colour? I have been almost blind to everything around me.

Today, though, as I look around the gardens, I can see so vividly the miraculous beauty in nature – so many luscious greens, vivid splashes of colour in the trees, bushes, flowers, ponds and the beautiful clear sky.

Somehow this is showing me that I need to get the colour back in my life. I need to find the beauty, happiness and laughter in every day. I need to allow myself to dance, act, walk, talk, learn and to allow my soul to feel joy and excitement again.

Today as I walked around the paths, looking for a message from heaven, looking at the surroundings of nature, I saw that some of the winding paths are a bit bare, barren and almost dead with dullness, but flowers and seeds have been planted, and in time they will blossom. I realise I need to plant new feelings of joy in my life and be patient. I feel like this garden of life has many bridges to cross and hills to climb but sometimes it's nice to stay with the familiar and take a walk on beautiful green grass.

As I sit here I can see a little cave in the corner of the garden – it has a roof and along the sides of the cave there is grass and some shrubs growing. I walked inside the cave and the air felt colder, but it was calm and peaceful. Inside, the old stone walls have little streams of water running down from the top – it looks like the walls are silently and gently crying. I feel like that inside, sometimes, but I am reminded that outside things are beginning to grow – outside things are blossoming and soon they will bloom with vibrant colour.

I came here wondering about my life and if I was on the right path, and suddenly, from just walking and spending time quietly in this garden alone with my thoughts and allowing all my senses to come alive, I seem to be able to think and see life clearly. I don't want to leave this magical space – the birds are singing, I can hear the gentle sound of the waterfall and I am surrounded by the wonders of nature. I am afraid if I leave this garden I won't feel this amazing feeling of safety and clarity.

Recording these thoughts in my journal makes them real, and it will mean that I won't forget them. I will be able to experience these feelings every time I read back over this entry. Sitting here writing and pondering my thoughts, I feel like I have the answers I need and the guidance I wanted.

'Each morning we are born again. What we do today is what matters most'

– Buddha

MONTHLY REVIEW

▸ This hypnosis relaxation will help you relax and unwind with the sounds and surroundings of the natural world.

▸ The free journal pages are for you to write freely about your journey – don't censor yourself and try to go with the flow of your train of thought.

▸ Why not try listening to your daily hypnosis relaxation while out in nature?

▸ If you find you are spending more time in nature this month, take inspiration and try using images of nature in your journal to add colour to the pages.

PROMPTS

What is your favourite season?

What is the most beautiful place in the world?

What element of nature speaks to you the most?

My Journal

'My ideas usually come not at my desk writing but in the midst of living.'
— Anais Nin

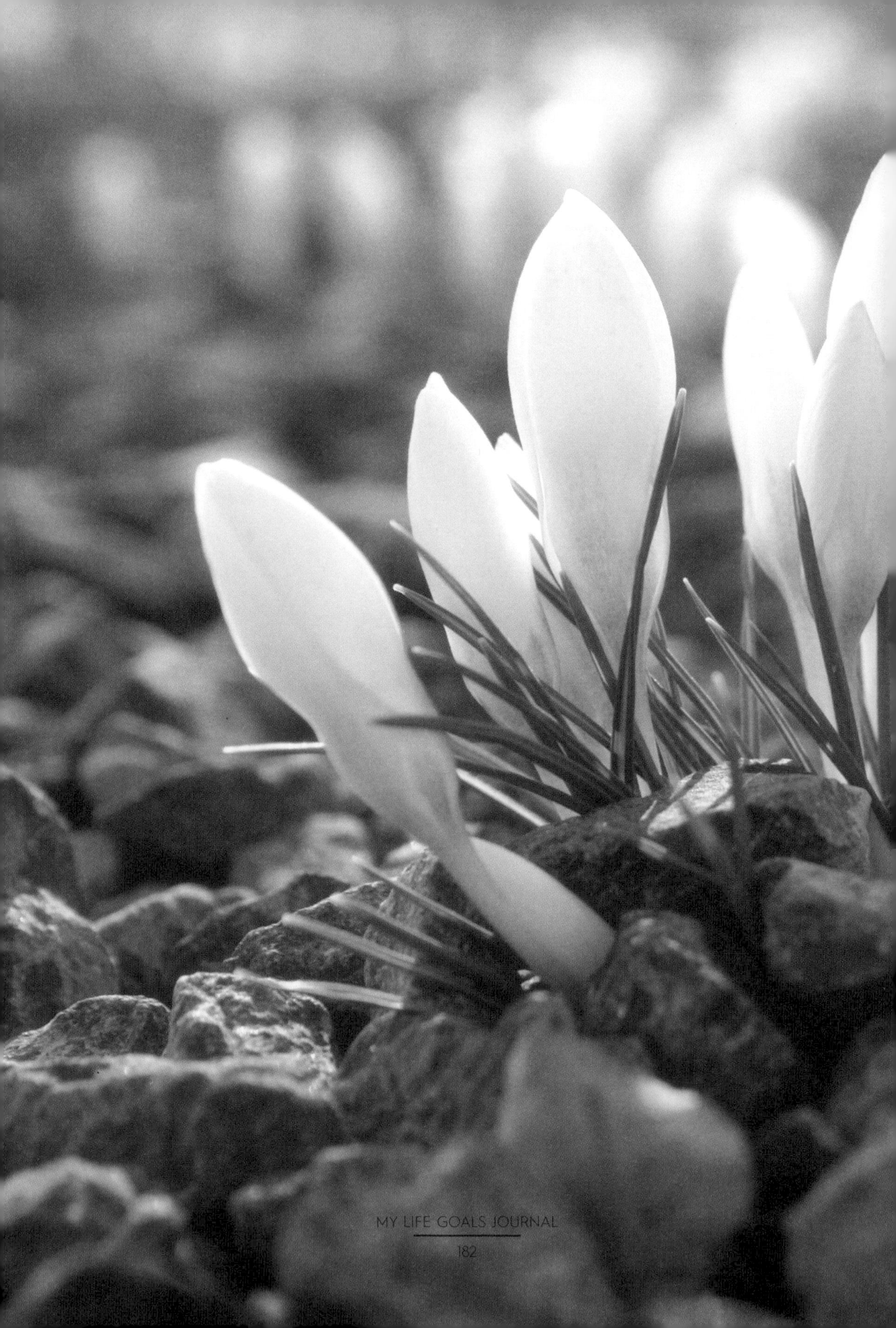

MONTH 8

Appreciation
of life

'I have chosen to be happy because it is good for my health'

– Voltaire

By now your journaling and monthly exercises should be establishing a secure foundation for a new and stronger you. Maybe it is time to focus on your life's **purpose** again and what **success** means to you.

The first step is to acknowledge and understand your worth and value. This wellness journey has brought you on a road of self-discovery and it is time to really **appreciate yourself** as a true blessing to the universe. This month, try using the following affirmation:

'Embrace and love your body – it is the most amazing thing you will ever own.'

Be mindful to stay focused on the positives. In your journal, get into the habit of writing down three things that went well each day, things you are grateful and happy for.

If you have been following the journal, you will by now have simplified many areas in your life and things should be flowing more easily. Even if you do not realise it, you are more centred in your sacred space. This is a good time to stretch yourself a little more and look to the future.

It is always a good exercise to take a moment to appreciate what brings you joy in every area of your life. On the next page you will find a useful chart that I use often to re-evaluate many different areas in my life. You can use this as a guide to write down what you are grateful for in each category and what you would like to attract too in that area of your life.

Take some time to consider all the wonderful blessings in your life as you think of them, and the feeling of gratitude will grow. You'll be amazed at how uplifting it is to turn your attention to the positive aspects of your life.

When you have a list completed of all the things you are thankful for, then dream big and imagine how you could sparkle even more and evoke even greater success into all areas of your life. In the column next to your list, detail what you want to attract or how you want to grow and develop in the coming months or year ahead.

AREA	I AM GRATEFUL FOR...
Career	
Home	
Family	
Friendships	
Health	
Recreation	
Fitness	
Education	
Personal growth	
Travel	
Fun	
Spiritual growth	
Community	

AREA	I WISH TO EXPAND AND SHINE BY ...
Career	
Home	
Family	
Friendships	
Health	
Recreation	
Fitness	
Education	
Personal growth	
Travel	
Fun	
Spiritual growth	
Community	

Have you heard of positive psychology?

When I was on my wellness journey I wanted to increase my happiness and well-being. I started reading about positive psychology – specifically a scientific study by Martin Seligman, who is credited as the father of positive psychology. In his book *Authentic Happiness* (2002), he explains that his journey towards this new field of study started off in an experiment about learned helplessness in dogs.

It proved to me that if I continued to expect a certain outcome with my health and wellness, I would get that outcome; but if I changed my expectations, my life would change. The more I learned about this form of scientific research the more I wanted to learn.

The field is founded on the belief that people want to lead meaningful and fulfilling lives, to cultivate what is best within themselves and to enhance their experiences of love, work and play.

We all want to be happier! In recent years so much of the research into happiness points to one main prescription: **gratitude**. In simple terms, saying two little words – **thank you** – has been proven to improve our well-being.

The Greater Good Science Center, based at the University of California, Berkeley, is unique in its commitment to both science and practice. They sponsor groundbreaking scientific research into social and emotional well-being and help people apply this research in their personal and professional lives. Scientists there have begun to chart a course of research aimed at understanding gratitude and the circumstances in which it flourishes or diminishes. They're finding that people who practise gratitude consistently report a host of benefits, including:

- Stronger immune systems and lower blood pressure
- Higher levels of positive emotions
- More joy, optimism and happiness
- Acting with more generosity and compassion
- Feeling less lonely and isolated

A 2005 study led by Martin Seligman found that the greatest contributing factor to overall happiness in life is how much gratitude we show. And a noticeable difference can be experienced with as little as three expressions each day – saying 'Thank you for …' just three times daily.

> A grateful mindset and appreciating the positive elements of life have the potential to improve your life dramatically.

DARE OF THE DAY

Say 'Thank you' often and with feeling today to as many people as you can. Sometimes it is the people closest to us that we forget to say those two simple words to – so make a point to go out of your way to say **thank you**! If you want to expand on this, you can choose to write a thank-you letter to someone who has done something nice for you in the past. Make sure to write the letter or card from the heart. Perhaps give someone you love in your life a little gift or present for no other reason than that you appreciate them and want to let them know.

DARE OF THE WEEK

You can increase your long-term happiness by almost 10 per cent with this simple daily habit from a study by Dr Martin Seligman. In the original study participants were asked to follow the instructions below. This week, try them for yourself.

- Every night for the next week, in your life goals journal, write down three things that went well today and why they went well. It is important that you have a physical record of your thoughts.

- The three things can be insignificant events, e.g. I ate my favourite dinner tonight, or significant events, e.g. my friend got a new job today!

- Next to each positive event, answer the question: 'Why did this happen?' For example, 'I took time to go shopping for all the ingredients to my favourite recipe' or 'My friend is talented and excellent at what she does and her talents have been recognised and she was the perfect person for the job.'

  Writing about why the positive events in your life happened may seem awkward at first, but please stick with it for one week. It will get easier.

Some things that went well today:

1. ....

2. ....

3. ....

Why did this happen?

1. ....

....

....

2. ....

....

....

3. ....

....

....

After one week, participants in Dr Seligman's study were 2 per cent happier than before, but in follow-up tests, their happiness kept on increasing – from 5 per cent at one month to 9 per cent at six months. All this, even though they were only instructed to journal for one week. Participants enjoyed the exercise so much that they just kept doing it on their own.

'We must find time to stop and thank the people who make a difference in our lives'

– John F. Kennedy

DARE OF THE MONTH

Make a gratitude board – this can be very powerful. Create a vision board that is all about the people, experiences and things in your life that make you feel grateful and thankful. Use a big board and include pictures or images that will spark happy memories. Leave it in your kitchen or bedroom where you will see it every day.

Creating a gratitude board will help you stay focused on the positives in your life and can lift you up when you're having a bad day.

If you don't want to make a board, you can use a page in your journal and fill it with visual references of all the things you are happy for. Also add images of things you hope to achieve.

ATTACH A PICTURE BELOW OF SOMETHING OR SOMEONE YOU ARE GRATEFUL FOR

'Reflect upon your present blessings, of which every man has plenty; not on your past misfortunes, of which all men have some'

– Charles Dickens

A DAY TO BE GRATEFUL FOR:
extract from my journal

Despite the pain, I choose to be happy and I feel blessed for so many positives in my life. Every day I feel so thankful for my wonderful family and I have to stay in this positive place and remind myself to count my blessings and focus on all the good in my life.

Today was a lovely day and a bit of a triumph for me personally. I am feeling very thankful for the amazing experiences that today brought. I went out for a playdate with our neighbour – we brought the little ones for an adventure and picnic on Killiney Hill. I forgot how beautiful the views are from up there: it was stunning. It was a lovely, clear day and I could see right across Dublin Bay, north to south: breath-taking. It was picture-postcard perfect.

The challenge for me personally was the climb. I was quite frightened seeing it, but I kept going and it was worth it for the view alone. I was in so much pain climbing the hill and coming down it was awkward too. I felt very unsteady on my feet and I really needed to concentrate so I didn't fall.

I know I should have said something but instead I kept going, probably just a little more quietly than normal. It's the old issue again of looking so well on the outside – I look healthy and normal and I feel like an attention seeker or a moaner if I flag that I am in pain. However, maybe I should be more honest about it.

On the upside, I am so grateful and I am so happy that I am getting out more and doing more, being braver, not fearing situations so much.

I am really trying to be gentler in my approach to my daily activities. It's amazing the difference in such a short period of time – things I would avoid are now places I go. Imagine that I would have missed that amazing experience if I hadn't challenged myself a little! So despite a little more pain I am so grateful for today's experience.

My sense of gratitude for the little things in life has really made me enjoy every experience so deeply and it has brightened up my days. I am going to bed tonight feeling so lucky and blessed. Thank you for my wonderful daughter, thank you for my lovely neighbours, thank you for all the natural beauty so close to where I live, thank you for my health and, yes, thank you for my body – despite the pain, my brain willed me on and I had a great day and conquered my fear and climbed a hill!

Thank you for today – it felt great.

'He is a wise man
who does not grieve
for the things which
he has not, but
rejoices for those
which he has'

– Epictetus

MONTHLY REVIEW

▸ This month's hypnosis relaxation will help you become more aware of gratitude and the power of daily blessings.

▸ How is your journal journey shaping up? Are you doing the work? If you are, then don't forget to be grateful for your commitment to this process. Remember, this month's theme is all about appreciation and that means appreciating yourself too.

▸ The daily hypnosis relaxations should be part of your routine and maybe you are exploring other types of hypnosis or relaxation now too.

▸ If you haven't done it already, maybe now is a good time to read back over your life goals journal and truly appreciate just how far you have come since the first entry.

PROMPTS

How is where you are in your life today different from when you started the journal?

Write about a person in your life, past or present, that you are grateful for and why:

What do you take for granted day to day and how can you show more appreciation?

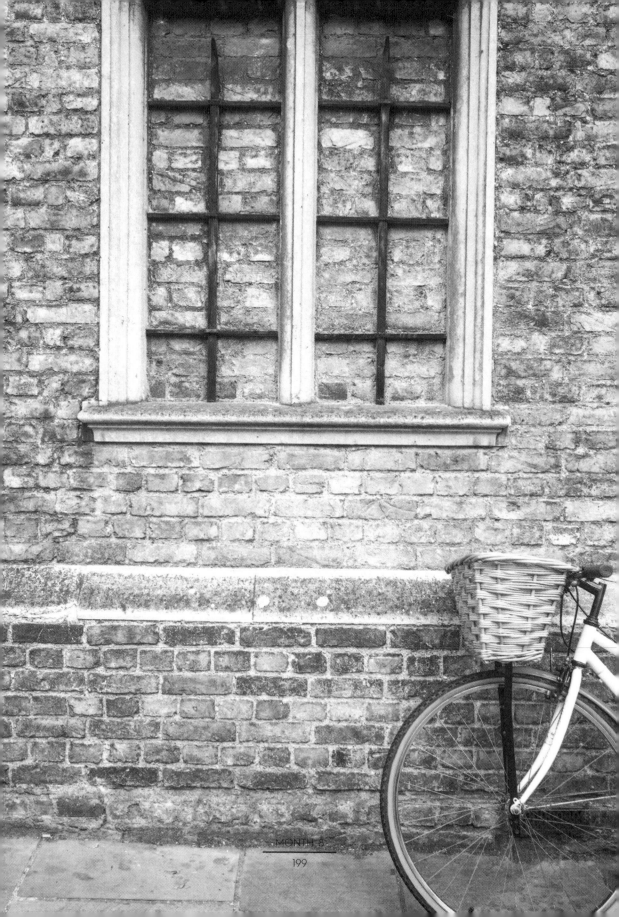

My Journal

'*Write what should not be forgotten.*'
– Isabel Allende

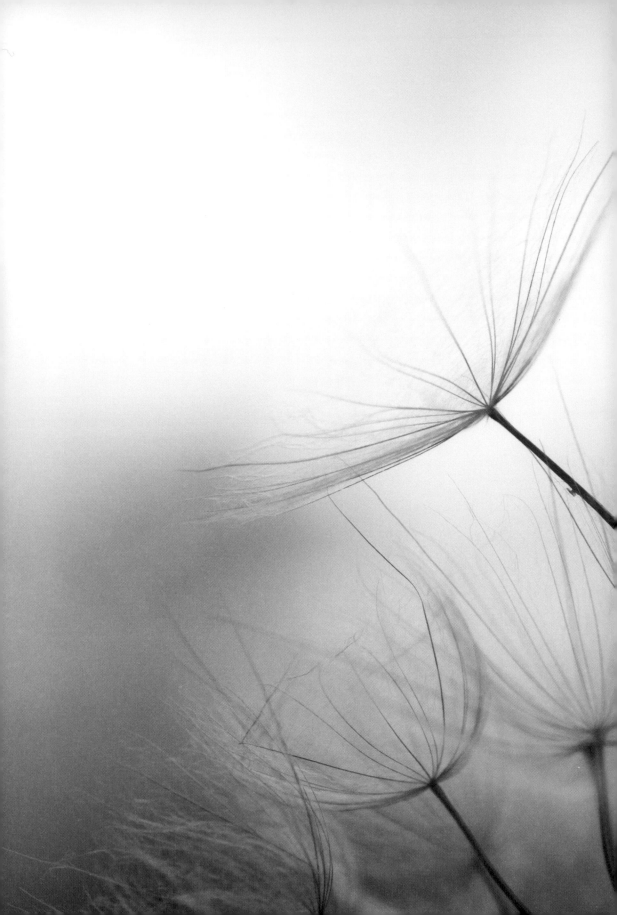

MONTH 9

Stress-free living

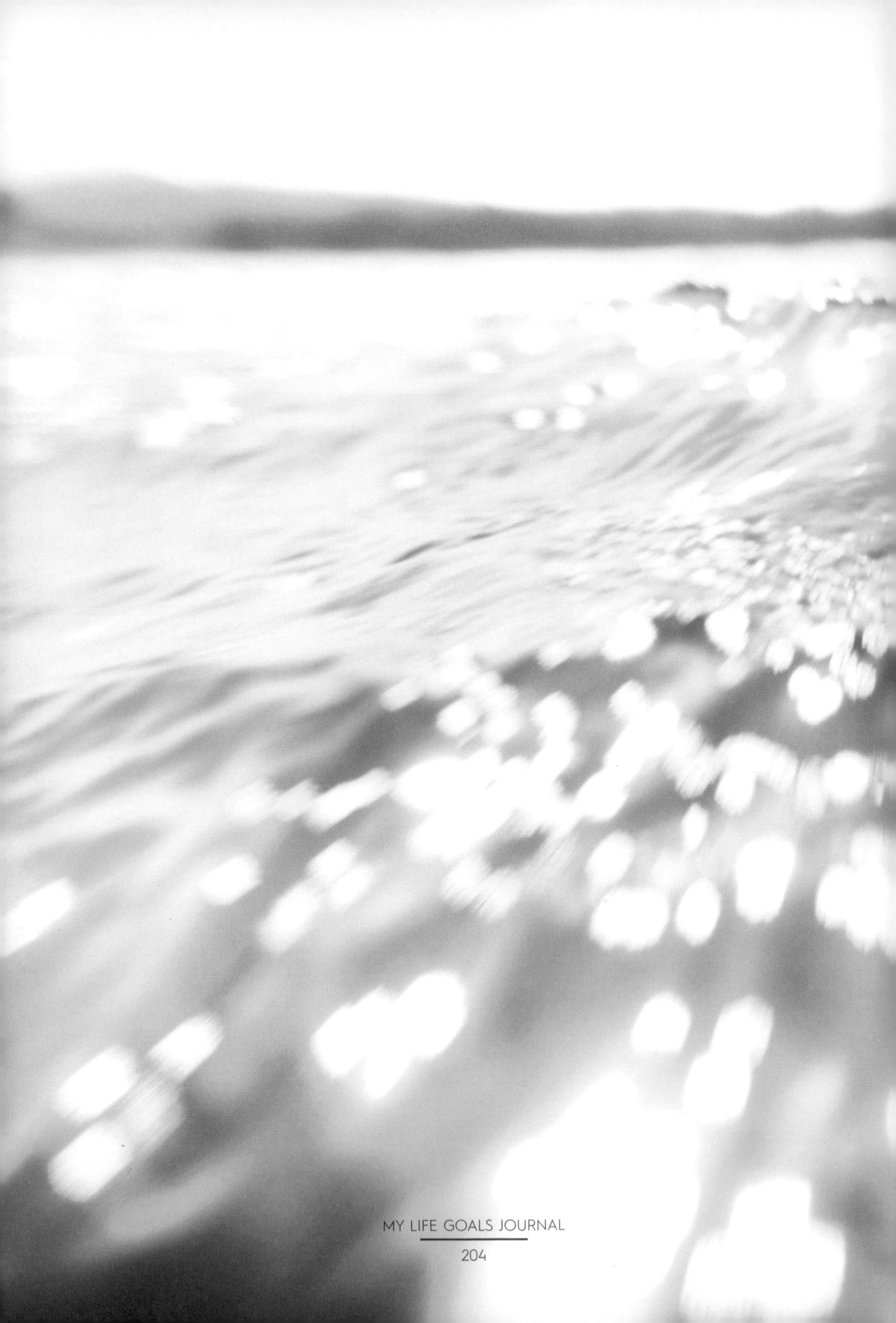

Everything in my life becomes more difficult to manage when I allow stress to take over. As we have learned so far on this journey, our minds are always working, processing our thoughts and opinions, and we know that if we believe statements and repeat or think them often, our subconscious minds will accept them to be true. Therefore the way we view situations and deal with them is essential for our wellness. Recognise the full value of how you react to stressful situations in your life.

> You can control your reactions and how you manage situations.

You will find this a little difficult if you have programmed yourself to look at things from a negative perspective, so this month make a conscious effort to look upon every situation in your life in a more **calm**, **confident** manner with an inner **trust** that things are unfolding perfectly for your higher good. Think positively – no matter how bad things might feel, everything has a positive aspect and often, when you look back at stressful situations, you will find that they caused you to change your route and that your new path brought you somewhere much better than you had originally planned to go.

The way you think can determine the outcomes of many situations in your life – are you choosing positive and beneficial thoughts or projecting negative and fear-based thoughts into your future?

The good news is that with persistence and focus you will find it easy to find positives in every situation. You will begin to acknowledge when you allow stressful thoughts to filter in and at that point you can start to say **stop**.

If you are still struggling to think positively during times of stress, here are some simple ways to help you change your viewpoint and begin to see the positives in every situation.

Just for today ...

Thinking **positively** is a very powerful habit to form – once your mindset and outlook change, something amazing happens: your view on the world around you changes and suddenly you remain **calm** and **at ease** even in difficult situations because you are always **expecting the best** possible outcome to manifest.

1. Every time you catch yourself thinking stressful or negative thoughts, **stop**, take a moment and imagine **deleting** that thought and replacing it with a positive one. There's no milk for your coffee? Delete the negative feelings of disappointment, pour a glass of water and think of how good it is to cleanse your system.

2. If you catch yourself catastrophising about the future and predicting a negative outcome or attaching failure to a situation that hasn't happened, **stop**, take a moment and begin to imagine yourself in the future and see that situation working out perfectly with the best possible outcome. **Visualise success** and allow that feeling to really sink in for a minute or two and then **believe** that to be true.

3. Monitor your language. If you hear yourself talking in a negative or pessimistic way, **stop**, take a moment and make a decision to keep your conversation **positive** or choose to say nothing at all. This will help you remain calm.

4. Surround yourself with positive people and live in a positive environment. It is easy to identify the people whose negative mindset can be draining and stressful to be around. Make a conscious effort to avoid these people. If you find you fall into stressful thought patterns in work **stop** and take note. Put a positive quote or uplifting image as your screen saver on your computer as a reminder to stay positive and **avoid** the **negative** nellies!

5. **Breathe** – centre yourself during moments of increased tension and allow yourself thirty seconds to **stop**. Begin by taking a deep breath – there is no greater gift we can give ourselves than the power of our breath connected to our consciousness. Breathing in slowly, think of things that bring you joy and, breathing out slowly, think of people or situations that fill you with love. Breathing in again, acknowledge that there are times when you need to just stop, and breathing out, admit that today you can choose your thoughts. Reach for positive ones. Taking another deep, healing breath in, and allowing the fresh air to balance your energies, then breathe out and consciously release stressful negative thoughts and energies. Spend a few seconds longer in this sacred space and then, when you're ready, continue on with your day.

6. Consciously smile more, and every time you smile remember that, from today, you are leaving negative stress-related thoughts behind you and forming new patterns towards positive thinking and behaviour. When in doubt, smile it out!

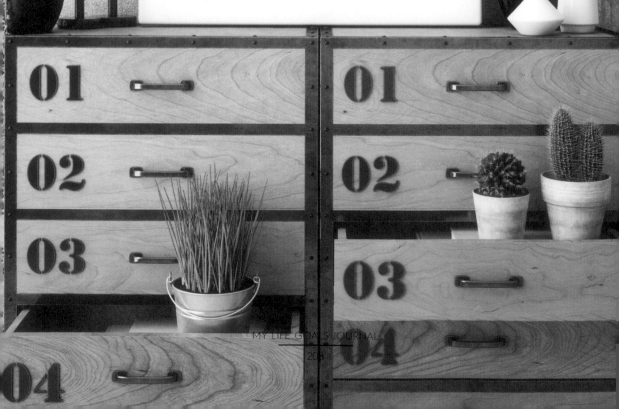

'Keep smiling,
because life is a
beautiful thing
and there's so
much to smile
about.'

– Marilyn Monroe

The wheel of life

Sometimes I find myself taking on additional stress when my life is out of balance – when I am not giving every area of my life equal measures of my time and attention. In today's busy world why do we find it so hard to get the balance right? It can be hard to juggle your career, money, health, social life, family, love, home and personal life. So if you feel like you're being pulled in any one direction, it is time to get your life aligned.

I **reconnect** with my inner navigation system to make sure I am on the right path with a simple **wheel of life** exercise, which I find very useful and effective in helping me deal with the stresses and strains of life.

When I am overwhelmed or out of balance and not pacing myself properly, I know it is time to take stock, anchor myself again and make sure I am going in the right direction.

The wheel of life is divided into categories that reflect different parts of your daily life and allow you to take a helicopter view of what's happening. You can then see if you are in balance or are spending too much time on one area or another. I find it very useful when I am faced with stressful situations, as it reminds me to identify what areas need more attention and helps me to see the **bigger picture** in my life.

Use the following steps to create your life wheel and assess your balance. Or use the wheel in this book and fill in your own sections.

THE WHEEL OF LIFE

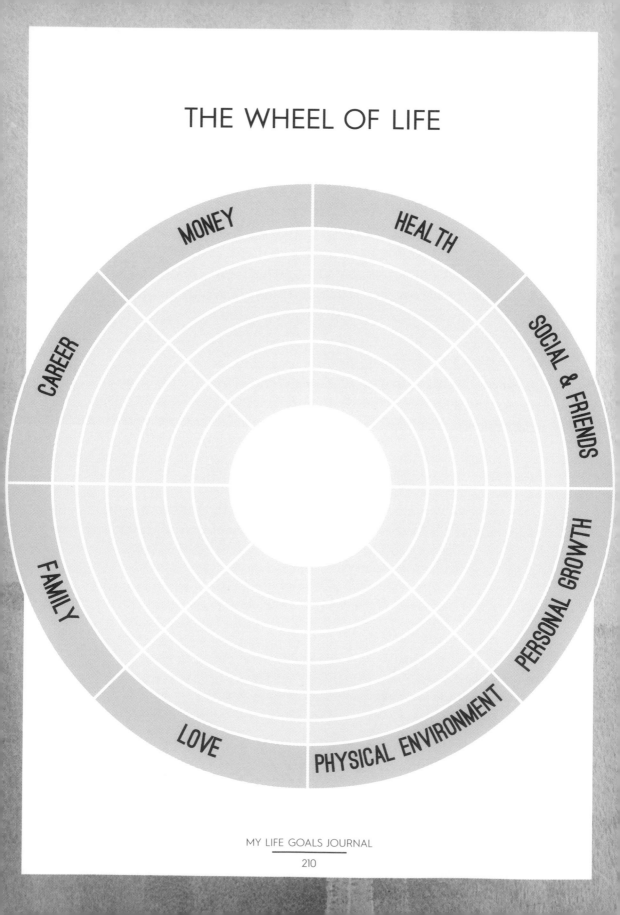

MONEY

HEALTH

CAREER

SOCIAL & FRIENDS

FAMILY

PERSONAL GROWTH

LOVE

PHYSICAL ENVIRONMENT

STEP 1

Think about the areas of life that are important to you. For our wheel here, I have chosen career, money, health, social and friends, family, love, physical environment and personal growth. If you don't feel that all of these categories apply to you, you can draw your own wheel in the blank pages at the end of this month's entry.

STEP 2

Reflect on each category and consider how much time and effort you give it. Using a scale of 0 (low) to 10 (high), write a number in each segment of the wheel to reflect the time currently devoted to this area in your life.

Some questions to ask yourself:

1. **Career:** Is your career where you want it to be by now? Are you heading in the right direction?

2. **Money:** Are you earning enough income to satisfy your current needs? Are you financially set up for future growth in wealth?

3. **Health:** How physically healthy are you? Are you satisfied with your level of fitness? Are you satisfied with your diet?

4. **Social and friends:** Are your friends supportive of you? Are you meeting friends and socialising enough? Are you having fun? Should you be spending more time meeting people and relaxing?

5. **Family:** Is your family supportive of you? Are you supportive of your family? Do you see your family enough and enjoy quality time together?

6. **Love:** Are you in love? Do you feel loved? How often do you express love to others?

7. **Physical environment:** Are you enjoying where you live? Do you live the way you want to live? Could you make better choices in the foods you buy? Are you conscious about the environment? Are you recycling?

8. **Personal growth:** Are you enjoying your life? How focused are you on personal growth? Are you satisfied with your direction? Are you trying new experiences and seeking to learn? Are you satisfied with your relationship with your spiritual being?

STEP 3

When you've answering the questions above and assessed each area of your life, think about your level of satisfaction and consider the amount of attention and focus you give each area. If an area is not currently a priority and you are not happy about that, you might give it a low score. If you focus too much attention on an area you might give it a high score.

Mark each score on the appropriate spoke of your life wheel.

STEP 4

Reflect on your wheel and see how balanced it is. Think about your time and how you could share it out more evenly to bring more happiness into your life in the areas that are lacking.

Are you completely out of balance in any area? You might notice that certain areas are interrelated – for instance, it can be difficult to go out socially if you don't have money, which may link to a low career score. If you begin to improve in one area, it will have a knock-on effect on other areas, so take time to see where you can redress the balance of your wheel. Ask yourself where you could make better choices with your time and energy.

STEP 5

Plan for change. Identify what areas need urgent attention and write down how you can regain balance in them. Make a commitment to take steps to change your wheel of life and decide how you will transform those areas that need positive change.

MY PLAN

1. Career:

....

....

....

2. Money:

....

....

....

3. Health:

....

....

....

4. Social and friends:

....

....

....

5. Family:

....

....

....

6. Love:

....

....

....

7. Physical environment:

....

....

....

8. Personal growth:

....

....

....

This is a brief insight into the wheel of life tool; there are many free online coaching sites that can be accessed to give you more support in using it. The key is to be aware of how balanced your life is: are you making good progress in some areas and not in others?

A low score doesn't mean you are unhappy – it simply represents an opportunity for growth and development.

If you find you need to make more headway in certain areas, take conscious steps to create opportunities and prioritise your time to focus on changes that will lead to a more fulfilling, successful and balanced life.

'The most important thing
is to enjoy your life – to be
happy – it's all that matters'

– Audrey Hepburn

DARE OF THE DAY

Take time today to write a letter to your future self and highlight what wonderful changes you want to manifest one year from now – or even project it further into the future, perhaps five or even ten years from now.

This can be fun but is also a powerful exercise. As you write about how well you will be doing in the future, you are engaging your subconscious mind and projecting those positive images of yourself to your consciousness.

Some tips, if you are finding this difficult:

▸ Start by writing today's date one year into the future.

▸ Congratulate your future self on one great goal accomplished in each area of your wheel of life exercise.

▸ Write a little more about your desired life and imagine what it is like to live life with your goals achieved. If you have more success in work, maybe you have more disposable income and you are using it for a great holiday, or you have upgraded your car. Think of what your future life is like and write about it in as much detail as possible.

▸ Once you are finished, lovingly remind yourself how proud you are of your achievements and sign your letter with your name and **today's** date.

DARE OF THE WEEK

This week, try a negative media detox. The media constantly bombard us with a lot of information about catastrophes, wars and other unhappy and negative events that we really have no control over. These bad-news stories can occupy our subconscious mind and begin to radiate negative thoughts to our own world and the community around us. It can become a steady stream of depressing messages that we can choose not to allow into our minds.

I tried this exercise and literally pulled the plug on all forms of media that report stories of disasters and pain. It was a difficult challenge, as I realised quickly I was constantly exposed to these stories every day – everywhere! But in doing so, I found I had more time on my hands, as I wasn't spending time reading or listening to reports of negative news. I also reminded myself how important music was for my soul. I listened to all my favourite tunes and it really uplifted my mood. I read only words of positivity or books I truly enjoyed and I slowly began to switch off negativity and tune into my own positive vibration and rhythm. The benefits of actively tuning out of toxic daily news reports are championed by various scientific studies. In simple terms: it is good for your health. Plus you will have more free time to focus on deeper thinking and a more mindful approach to daily life.

DARE OF THE MONTH

Now that you have made your wheel of life and are experienced in using it, develop a wheel of life for specific areas like goal setting or time management. For example, if you find you don't have enough time in the day to finish tasks, maybe try to write all your goals for the day into a wheel, give each task a specific amount of time you want to focus on it and try to stick to that. At the end of the day you can review it and score the actual time spent at a task and see if you are out of balance. This is a useful tool to review things in a visual way.

Use the wheel of life exercise to identify what you want to focus on, your goals. It is an adaptable tool that can be used to visualise what you want to manifest in the future.

WRITING A LETTER TO MY FUTURE SELF:
extract from my journal

I have started a new habit: I am keeping my gratitude habit going every night, but I have started also to write one page of things I am grateful for that haven't even happened yet. I started it last week and it felt very uplifting – it was like I was projecting some positivity into the future and planting seeds of change into my mind to attract these changes. I've kept doing it and now I am looking forward to it, oddly, every night. I was inspired by a piece I read online about writing a letter to your future self so I decided to give that a go too:

    Dear Andrea,

    I want to start by saying thank you for all your hard work – you have manifested a steady stream of abundance which is reaching you every day in many ways. I am so grateful for all the positive changes you have embraced and all the joy, love and health that fills your daily life because of your new habits.

    You have begun new fitness routines, which are adding to your overall well-being, and your dedication to your wellness is benefiting not only you but all the family too.

    I am so happy and proud of you for all the work you have put into feeling well and for following your own healing instincts on your pain-management plan. It is not easy, no day is, but you are filled with energy and vitality and are using this to explore new avenues for work that are truly fulfilling and fun. You are blessed to have so much financial reward for all your work efforts – you are paid fairly and promptly for your dedication and commitment to everything you work at.

    Andrea, because you radiate positivity and health from your heart, you attract wonderful people into your life and you have brilliant friends to support you, and who you support, and who encourage your new lifestyle choices and decisions.

    I am so grateful that the universe constantly keeps bringing great surprises into your life and things seem to flow easily and effortlessly for you in all areas. I am so thankful for the excellent exam results you have received and all the wonderful mentors and teachers who have helped you on your learning journey. You now have endless opportunities to share your new-found knowledge with others and it will help people greatly and bring you immense satisfaction.

Finally, Andrea, well done for taking time to love yourself and all those around you. You are blessed with a healthy daughter, a supportive and loving husband and a great companion in Dash. In time your family will grow and the love you share will continue to expand. Every day is an opportunity to grow more in love and gratitude.

Keep doing what you're doing.
Love, Andrea x

'Life isn't about finding yourself. Life is about creating yourself'

– George Bernard Shaw

MONTHLY REVIEW

- This hypnosis relaxation is perfect for unwinding and destressing a cluttered mind.

- Are your journal pages filling up easily and effortlessly? Maybe some months are easier than others – maybe that is something you could review?

- Relaxation is a great way to release stress and the extended hypnosis on my website for this month's theme can be used to help you become more calm and balanced.

- When life's challenges seem overwhelming, journaling is a great way to help put anything that is causing you stress into perspective.

PROMPTS

Write about your emotions – what makes you happy, angry, fearful, stressed, sad?

Do you have a particular worry? Use the journal to brainstorm solutions to that problem

_____

_____

_____

_____

_____

_____

_____

What have you gained from past challenges? Remind yourself of lessons learned:

_____

_____

_____

_____

_____

_____

Write a letter to your future self

Dear Me ...

_____

_____

_____

_____

_____

_____

_____

_____

_____

_____

_____

_____

_____

_____

My Journal

'Journaling is like whispering to one's
self and listening at the same time.'
                    – Mina Murray, Dracula

MONTH 10

Stillness and sleep

'Do not dwell in the past,
do not dream of the future,
concentrate the mind on the
present moment'

– Buddha

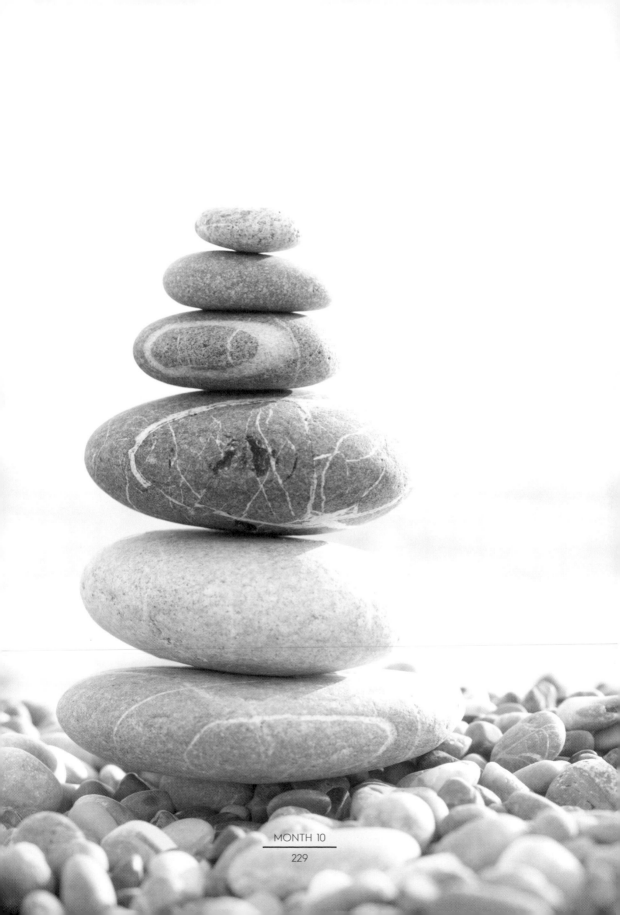

Learning to be still

In order to discover your true essence and life purpose, take time to **rest** your body and soul. Find, understand and use **stillness** and **solitude** to allow wonderful breakthroughs to occur in your subconscious.

I have had many dark moments when my health challenges overwhelmed me but on those days I realised it is during a season of isolation that the caterpillar gets its wings. I have learned to embrace solitude and use it to recharge.

It was a big lesson for me to learn that it is OK to rest and I now enjoy the practice of active relaxation. You can too by listening to the hypnosis relaxations listed at the end of each month in this journal. As you listen to them you are resting your mind and body while still benefiting from all the subconscious positive suggestions.

In today's society we want and demand everything right now. We are constantly on the go, rushing from meeting to meeting, trying to make deadlines, emailing, sending texts, on social media, always thinking, always talking, always connected, and for me, I found I was always **on**!

I couldn't switch off and I felt if I wasn't connected I was missing something. I was. I was losing connection with myself, my body, my mind and my true essence. My wellness journey forced me to embrace stillness and it took a long time to learn what that really meant. For me, it wasn't just about not being connected to my mobile device: it was about giving myself space to relax and to breathe, to focus on my progress.

Think of your life and ask yourself when in your daily life do you allow time to embrace being still?

TRY THIS EXERCISE

Read the examples then fill in your own answers – add a time or place to the words and allow these emotions and moments to happen.

I am **tranquil** when I allow myself to
have a long bath.

I am **quiet** when I am reading
an enjoyable book.

I am **calm** when I am listening
to my relaxations.

I am **still** when I am meditating in nature.

I am **gentle** when I am spending time
with my dog.

I am **placid** when I am surrounded
by those I love.

I am **restful** when I relax on the couch
after a long walk.

I am **serene** when I indulge in a massage
or healing treatment.

I am **hushed** when I listen to
my favourite music.

I am **peaceful** when I am alone in prayer.

I am **tranquil**

I am **quiet**

I am **calm**

I am **still**

I am **gentle**

I am **placid**

I am **restful**

I am **serene**

I am **hushed**

I am **peaceful**

Schedule quiet time for yourself

It was my connection to my faith that allowed me to truly experience what it means to be still, but everyone must find their own way forward. Sometimes not doing anything is more **powerful** than taking action and this is a big lesson to learn. When we approach our daily challenges from a place of stillness, we are better able to see the bigger picture – we are more able to be tranquil, quiet, calm, still, gentle, placid, restful, serene, hushed or peaceful.

'Be still and know that I am God', Psalms 46:10, is a phrase I hold onto when I need to find quiet.

Try to make it your intention to connect to your inner 'still' place.

HOW DOES BEING STILL AFFECT THE QUALITY OF YOUR AWARENESS?

Start to notice the profound relationship between **outer** and **inner stillness**. Paying attention in this way is part of being mindful, and it is the first step in learning the subtle dynamics of **awareness**. Meditation is one of the most powerful ways to harness and train your awareness, and the more still you are able to become, the deeper your capacity for meditation.

I have adopted my own meditation methods, which involve being still and becoming aware of my breath. You can find many different types of meditations online, but for now, just try to become aware of being still for a short time each day and become **aware** of what you experience during this time. Write about it in your journal and notice how you enjoy the process.

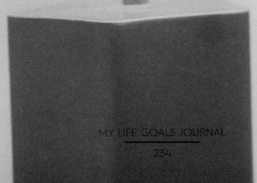

'Sleep is the best
meditation'

– Dalai Lama

Good sleep hygiene

On average a person sleeps for eight hours a day, which means that an average person will sleep for 229,961 hours in their lifetime – one-third of our lives. Far from being wasted time, from the moment we slide into unconsciousness, a whole raft of functions takes place to make sure that we get optimal benefit from our nightly rest.

According to the National Sleep Foundation, most healthy adults need seven to nine hours of sleep a night. However, some individuals are able to function without sleepiness or drowsiness after as little as six hours' sleep. Others can't perform at their peak unless they've slept ten hours.

We all know that a good night's rest makes you feel better but the importance of sleep goes way beyond just boosting your mood. Sleep plays an important role in your physical health. For example, sleep is involved in the healing and repair of your heart and blood vessels; ongoing sleep deficiency is linked to an increased risk of heart disease, kidney disease, high blood pressure, diabetes and stroke.

As well as being good for our health and our ability to perform at our best, sleep also is good for our relationships. At the 2013 Society for Personality and Social Psychology (SPSP) annual meeting, scientists from UC Berkeley presented new research suggesting that inadequate sleep can impair our ability to appreciate our partners and loved ones, which can lead to stress and tension in relationships. The SPSP reports that less sleep means fewer feelings of gratitude and higher levels of selfishness, both of which can make a partner feel unacknowledged and underappreciated.

BEDTIME HABITS TO OPTIMISE OUR SLEEP

I first heard the term **sleep hygiene** on my pain-management course and, contrary to the images the name conjures up, it has nothing to do with clean bedsheets or your washing routine. In fact it relates to the habits and practices that are conducive to sleeping well on a regular basis.

When you have chronic pain, getting a regular night's sleep is like the Holy Grail – an elusive goal that often is impossible. I learned that I could set myself up for success with a few simple tips and tricks.

There are many books about this topic but these are some of the changes I made that helped me along the way.

1. Create the right **mood** and set the scene. Turn your bedroom into a sleep-inducing environment. Try to make it dark, relaxing, quiet and peaceful. For me, this meant switching off the TV and listening to my relaxations. This was a big change for me, but it worked and I seemed to relax more.
2. Make **healthier choices** before bed: avoid caffeine, alcohol, nicotine and other chemicals that interfere with sleep. Eat lightly in the evening, as going to bed with a full stomach won't help.
3. Keep your internal clock set with a **consistent sleep schedule**. Try to establish a soothing pre-sleep routine – this could be having a nice bath or reading a book or meditating. Whatever you choose, keep it consistent and relaxing.
4. Try to **avoid daytime napping**. This seems obvious but because I wasn't sleeping at night I would rest during the day and this just made it more difficult to sleep at night. If you do need to nap, try to limit your snooze session to thirty minutes, and give yourself at least four hours between the nap and when you plan to go to bed properly.
5. Keep note of your **sleeping habits** in your journal. This can help establish a routine – plus, if you identify that you have a problem falling asleep at night, it can be helpful if you need to share your sleep patterns with your doctor. Insomnia can be a serious issue that may need medical intervention so don't be afraid to seek advice from your GP.

THE IMPORTANCE OF DREAMS

As well as all the restorative functions that kick in when we sleep, it is also our time to dream – and getting plenty of sleep is the first step to good dream recall.

Dreams are responsible for many of the greatest inventions of mankind, including Larry Page's idea for Google, Tesla's alternating current generator and Elias Howe's design for the sewing machine.

Dreams are responsible not only for great inventions and great works of art but also for **recharging** our creativity. There is a whole subculture of people practising what is called **lucid** or **conscious dreaming**, which enables them to tap into the power of their dreams and find hidden messages.

Understanding **your dreams** opens a **doorway** to your **subconscious.**

———

Is something bothering you that is preventing you from moving forward in an aspect of your life? This will take shape in your subconscious mind while you are asleep – if you can **unlock your dreams** you can understand your relationships with other people and events and tackle issues that may not have presented themselves clearly in your conscious world.

If you are well rested it will be easier to focus on your goal of recalling dreams. There is mounting scientific evidence to suggest that dreaming is good for us. Rubin Naiman, a sleep and dream expert from the clinical faculty of the Arizona Center for Integrative Medicine, says, 'Good dreaming contributes to our psychological well-being by supporting healthy memory, warding off depression, and expanding our ordinary limited consciousness into broader, spiritual realms.'

In the dream state your brain isn't bound by the same logical rules as it is during waking life. While dreaming you create **new connections** and different associations – this actually allows you to create new neural pathways in your brain. **The result: enhanced creativity and increased ability to solve problems.**

So getting a good sleep is not only good for your health: it is also good for your ability to dream. Longer sleep periods will lead to longer dream periods; we all dream every night, about one dream period every ninety minutes.

People who say they never dream simply don't remember their dreams. Dreams occur when our bodies are in the sleeping stage known as REM, which stands for Rapid Eye Movement, sleep. The body is at rest, but the mind is active with dreams. If you don't get enough sleep at night, or your sleep is interrupted a lot, you get less REM sleep and fewer dreams. Most people need between seven and nine hours of sleep every night to achieve the right amount of rest. People who sleep less than six hours have difficulty remembering dreams because longer, more vivid dreams take place later in the sleeping cycle. You may have more than one dream during a REM (dream) period. The whole area of dream recall is fascinating and there are many books and plenty of scientific research on the subject if you want to find out more.

'You are never too old to set another goal or to dream a new dream'

– C.S. Lewis

Here are a few tips to help you remember your dreams.

1. Stop burning the midnight oil and plan to be into bed **early**. Consider starting a new sleep routine with an earlier start.
2. Relax and **unwind** before you go to bed. Make it your intention to calm your mind and body before bedtime. Try meditating or using the self-hypnosis counting technique to free your mind from stressful thoughts.
3. Set your **intention**: think about what question you would like answered during your dream. Think about the problem that is concerning you right before you fall asleep – don't look for solutions: just allow your mind to process the thoughts that you are seeking a solution to, and your dreams may offer more insights regarding the problem at hand.
4. Put your **journal** and **pen** or pencil within easy reach of your bed. Before you go to sleep, make sure your journal is open to a blank page so you don't have to search for one when you wake up to jot down your dreams.
5. Make a **conscious decision** to remember your dreams. Before you go to sleep, write down your intention of remembering your dreams vividly and easily. You've got a better chance of remembering your dreams if you really **want** to remember them. Use an affirmation to tell yourself that you're going to remember your dreams and concentrate on recalling your dream when you wake.
6. Get into the habit of **recounting** your dream as soon as you wake up. Research suggests you only remember the last dream you had before waking, so as soon as you are aware you are awake, immediately begin to describe your dream. Avoid moving or rolling over – stay in the same position and try to remember as much about your dream as possible before you think about anything else. When you have it clear in your mind, pick up your journal and get writing.
7. **Record** your dream in your journal. Jot down as much detail as possible, starting with a basic outline that includes such things as the location of the dream, the basic plot, the characters, the overall emotion of the dream. If you can remember any dialogue, you may want to write it down first, as words in dreams are easily forgotten. Record everything you can, even if you can only remember one image. As you get the basics down, more of the dream may come to you.

8. How did the dream make you feel? This is important too, so write down how you're feeling when you wake up. The **emotions** you experience in a dream can reveal a lot. If you wake up anxious or elated, ask yourself why. Consult a dream dictionary and try to see what explanation it gives for the themes and feelings you experienced in your dream and write that beside your account of it.

You will find after some practice it becomes easier and your dreams may offer a great insight into what is going on inside your subconscious – try it!

RECORD TONIGHT'S DREAMS:

'Without leaps of imagination or dreaming, we lose the excitement of possibilities. Dreaming, after all, is a form of planning'

– Gloria Steinem

stillness when I breathe. Earlier this evening, I found silently saying a soothing word helped my mind to become more at ease. It helped to keep me from jumping ahead with thoughts of what I needed to be doing or worrying about cleaning my house and other mad thoughts that often jump into my psyche.

So overall it was a mixed day with the meditation. It probably won't be as easy as I thought, and like all things it might take me a while to perfect it, but I will work at it and I feel already that just recognising how little I practise peace and stillness through my day is a valuable lesson.

Pick

Wh
hor

'The future belongs to those who believe in the beauty of their dreams'

– Eleanor Roosevelt

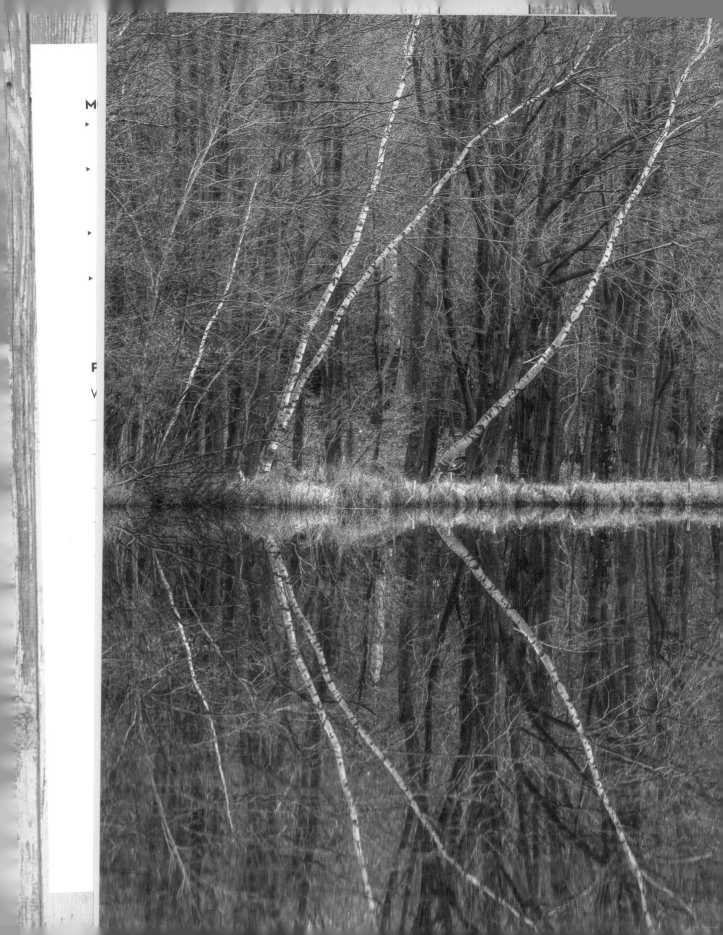

MONTH 11

Surrender and let go

'It is not in the stars to hold our destiny but in ourselves'

– William Shakespeare

Time to let go

This month, make a conscious effort to let go. Relinquish your grip on someone, something or a situation that no longer serves you – allow the act to set you free. Let go of fear about the future, let go of fear about security, let go of hurtful habits, let go of any expectations that are holding you back and set yourself free.

Take some time now to honour this month's intention and let go with love of whatever needs to be released – write a list of the things that come to mind. Do you need to drink less, stop biting your nails, end a difficult relationship? Think of the things that are preventing you from reaching your goals and hampering you from achieving your dreams.

LET GO LIST

1.

2.

3.

4.

5.

6.

7.

8.

9.

10.

Writing down things that no longer have a place in your life can be emotional so **acknowledge** and **honour** your feelings.

Take all the time you need to grieve and understand that this is part of a process of renewal. You may not feel happy about letting go, but if deep down you feel it is the right thing to do, take that step this month. If you do begin to experience **happiness** at the prospect of change, don't feel guilty! Whatever emotions you have are right for you at this point. Just acknowledge you are **letting go** of toxic people or situations in your life. This is a major step on the road to becoming happier and more content.

Facing your fears

According to Albert Einstein, the definition of insanity is 'doing the same thing over and over again and expecting different results'.

Now is the time to give up fear and live your dreams. You can't control everything in life, but you can control your own thoughts, so trust now and have faith that everything is going to work out. All is well: you are safe and secure and have let go a little and allowed your positive mind and abundant expectation to release the good that life has to offer.

Fear can paralyse you, and most people cling to their fears because it's part of who they are.

> **Make a point now to face your fears and transcend them.**

Allow yourself to think of all the things, people or situations that bring up fear-based thoughts.

It might be hard at first but pinpoint all the things that cause you fear and uncertainty. The first step in facing your fears is accepting them and acknowledging them. Take time to identify what fears hold you back at this moment – you may have a fear about your body, career, finances, relationships or even success and reaching goals and dreams.

Be fearless and identify your fears.

WHAT ARE YOU REALLY SCARED OF?

1. ....

....

2. ....

....

3. ....

....

4. ....

....

5. ....

....

6. ....

....

7. ....

....

8. ....

....

9. ....

....

10. ....

....

It is time to release your fears. Accept it is time to stop holding onto what makes you sad or hurt and reach for things that bring you joy and happiness.

Now – using the columns in the blank table – write two lists. Starting with the first fear you wrote down earlier, write a list of any anxieties you hold relating to that – what are the worst things that can happen? You don't succeed; you experience shame or embarrassment? Whatever you feel is the worst-case scenario, write it down and then think about whether this is really true.

In the second column, write out all the good things that could manifest if you challenge your fears. Think of all the things you stand to gain if you go after your goals or dreams – like feelings of satisfaction, fulfilment and self-growth!

This is a great exercise to help you face your fear – instead of thinking of something bad that could happen, you think of something **positive**.

What's a positive outcome to your fear? If you're thinking about public speaking, imagine yourself being wildly successful instead of failing horribly.

FEAR	THE WORST THING THAT COULD HAPPEN	THE BEST POSSIBLE OUTCOMES
Public Speaking	Stress Failure Embarrassment	Success Pride Achievement Acceptance

FEAR	THE WORST THING THAT COULD HAPPEN	THE BEST POSSIBLE OUTCOMES

By challenging your fears you soon will realise that many are created by your own imagination – and often your **thoughts** about what you fear are a lot scarier than that fear is in **reality**.

When you take action and face your fears, they become weaker because you realise that reality isn't nearly as bad as your imagination.

Learning to deal with fear is all about putting your negative thoughts in **perspective**. We tend to focus too much on the negative, so by looking at all the options, you can see that you're making a big deal of nothing. There are so many things that can happen that it's impossible for you to predict, so try to **stay grounded** and keep your thoughts rooted in realistic, positive outcomes.

I believe we all go through things for a reason. That includes the fears we have. So ask yourself: what are my feelings of fear trying to tell me? Ask what the purpose of them is. Ask your heart, God, the universe or whatever you feel comfortable with.

What are your fears trying to tell you?

Overcoming fear and learning the lessons that come out of that is part of our life journey. We have much to learn along the way, but remember, no matter what happens, **life goes on**. We continue to learn from every situation, even failure – sometimes our failures can be our biggest lessons – and even when we fail, life goes on. Thomas Edison said, 'I have not failed. I've just found 10,000 ways that won't work.'

Ask yourself: **is my fear genuine**? Explore the roots of your fears. If a similar fear is repeated in different situations, ask yourself if it is related to a deeper issue. This may require some meditation or deeper thought and exploration with a counsellor.

Look inside and ask yourself how the fear started – when did it happen? Did this fear manifest when you were younger? Getting to the root cause of the fear and setting it free can be very **healing**.

Remember that the only thing that matters is that you listen to yourself and be true to your inner voice. Whatever fears you're facing, you can overcome them and transcend to a better place in your heart and mind.

WHAT HAVE YOU LEARNED ABOUT YOUR FEARS?

'Ever tried.
Ever failed.
No matter.
Try Again.
Fail again.
Fail better.'
– Samuel Beckett

Surrendering control

Feelings of needing to control everything are rooted in fear. Surrender literally means to **stop fighting** – can we choose to stop resisting and pushing against our reality? Attempting to control our surroundings means we limit possibilities. As we surrender we begin to open up to all options, especially those beyond what we can see. Just because we can't see a solution doesn't mean the perfect one isn't just around the corner, hidden from our vison. Are you willing to truly release and let go?

Letting go and **trusting** in life to bring us great blessings is not an action of weakness but an action of great strength. We need to begin to believe that things are meant to come with divine timing and sometimes it is time to let go in our lives.

A big lesson in life is acknowledging that you have **limitations** – you can only do what you can do. Tell yourself that you are doing the very best you can at this moment and that is perfect for right now.

You have everything inside of you necessary to deal with anything life brings your way. Release old patterns and beliefs about your ability to cope, loosen the grip on the past and stop trying to control the future. Delete any notions from your mind of how things are 'supposed' to be and instead decide to just 'be' in this moment fully and 'be' present.

TRY THIS EXERCISE

Take time to be mindful in this moment, to let go and surrender. Centre yourself for this mindful moment.
Start by taking a deep breath:

- Breathing in harmony …

- And breathing out harmony …

Take another deep breath:

- Breathing in happiness …

- And breathing out happiness …

Make a conscious effort now to let go of negative thoughts, associations or fears. Take a deep breath in and on your exhale let go of fear about the future:

- Let go of fear about security ...

- Let go of hurtful habits and expectations ...

- Let go of someone or something that no longer serves you – allow the act to set you free ...

Honour this intention and let go, with love, whatever needs to be released:

- Breathing in happiness ...

- Breathing out harmony ...

Spend a few seconds longer breathing in happiness and harmony, and when you're ready, open your eyes.

Practise this mindful meditation for two to three minutes any time you have a space to fill in your day. Say goodbye to old energy and allow new seeds of possibility to grow and blossom.

SELF-REFLECTION EXERCISE

It is important to make time for careful introspection in order to learn more about yourself and define what is important for you. It is a great way to gain clarity about your life choices, but it takes some considered thought and time. The word **reflection** means 'to think about something' and **self** is defined by 'one's own experiences'.

No one else can self-reflect on your life – only you!

Ask yourself, in the various areas of your life:

1. What have I learned?

....

....

....

....

2. What am I grateful for?

3. What do I still want to achieve?

4. What do I want to release?

5. What do I want to focus on?

....

....

....

....

....

....

6. What have I done really well achieving balance in?

....

....

....

....

....

....

7. Why do I believe in myself?

....

....

....

....

....

....

I TRUST ALL
IS WELL AND
THIS WILL
MANIFEST.

'You don't have to see the whole staircase, just take the first step'

– Martin Luther King, Jr

DARE OF THE DAY

Take action today to reach beyond your fears and closer to your dreams and goals.

It doesn't have to be time-consuming – reach out to a friend, send an email for a job, make that important call, book onto that course. Pitching one idea or writing one page can be the catalyst you need to spark massive change in your life. Whatever it is you do, let it be enough and trust you have done enough!

Today I will move closer to my dream by:

....

....

....

....

....

DARE OF THE WEEK

When you're gripped by fear and anxiety, it's usually because you're stepping out of your **comfort zone**. Take some time this week to do something that stretches your limits and scares you just a little bit. In taking the challenge to confront your fear, you're already a winner.

Example – join a social group.

DARE OF THE MONTH

One of the quickest and most effective ways to overcome fear is to take a single, bold step forward in the direction of your dreams – to prove to yourself that you are willing to do what it takes.

You have a brand new month ahead to achieve your ultimate goal. Release your fear, dare to dream the impossible and go, go, go.

This month tackle one of your biggest fears and believe in your ability to follow your own path and trust that you are going in the right direction.

For example, learn something new, ask for a salary increase or start a blog. Whatever you do, make a leap into the unknown and trust it is for your higher good!

'Nothing is impossible
– the word itself says
I'M-POSSIBLE'

– Audrey Hepburn

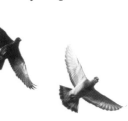

HOW I EMBRACED FEAR:
extract from my journal

*I didn't realise how much fear I have about my health. I have learned so much in recent months but I actually have so much more to learn. I have to somehow make peace with my health and stop allowing it to affect my future. I suddenly realised today that maybe I would like to have another child in time to come, but I am so worried about my health degenerating that I have projected that into my destiny and I am worrying unnecessarily about something that hasn't even happened. It is totally irrational and yet I am afraid for what tomorrow will bring. This needs to **stop**.*

It all became clear after my check-up appointment with my GP earlier today. We had a good chat about how I am doing and where I am in my progression with my medication and pain management and I am doing really well. I am off almost all my medication and only now is it possible for me to think about getting pregnant.

We discussed it and just the thought and conversation about the whole area of having another child made me very emotional and suddenly all my secret fears about the future began to bubble to the surface. So I cried and started to tell her a list of things I was worried about: further nerve damage, new pains, loss of control and function and other things that I have been avoiding, and it was actually really good to get everything off my chest. I am filled with fear that I may not be able to get pregnant and then, if I did, would I be able to manage the pregnancy and caring for another child?

After much discussion I feel better, and we decided to tackle the matter when I am fully off my medication – we can look into options and specialists then, which is the right plan of action.

However it has made me really focus on the whole concept of fear and projecting unpleasant feelings of distress and dread into my future. Fear is never a good thing, but it is so important to recognise and acknowledge feelings of fear before they take hold. I am going to chat to David about the whole subject and try to work through how I am feeling. I feel I need to write out a list of everything I am frightened of and then work from that and talk about everything and release my anxieties. I think once I realised that everybody feels anxious about the possibility of getting pregnant, it helped me, and knowing I have the support of a great GP and brilliant doctors, already my mind is more at ease and that feeling of terror is gone. It is amazing how just writing about emotions and talking about things can really help change the energy of the situation and put things into perspective.

I think I am going to do some breathing exercises and find my sacred space and say thank you for the great GP I have. I am very lucky and I know I have so much to look forward to.

'We are awakened
to the profound
realisation that
the true path to
liberation is to let
go of everything'

– Jack Kornfield

MONTHLY REVIEW

- ‣ This hypnosis relaxation will help you let go of old habits or situations that are holding you back or stopping you from reaching your life's purpose.

- ‣ As we near the end of the journal journey, it is a great time to review and reflect on how you enjoyed the experience.

- ‣ Head over to the website to listen to this month's hypnosis relaxation, which will help you face your fears and create the life you dream of.

- ‣ Don't be afraid to just write down words that inspire you or lyrics from a song that has a special meaning – it's your personal journal: no one is judging.

PROMPTS

Define what you believe to be success and what you consider to be failure:

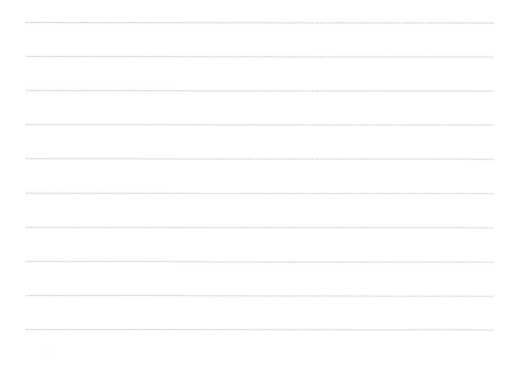

Remember a time when you experienced failure. What happened? What did you learn?

_____

_____

_____

_____

_____

_____

_____

Write a note to someone or something that made you fearful in the past:

_____

_____

_____

_____

_____

_____

_____

My Journal

'This one step – choosing a goal and sticking to it – changes everything.'

– Scott Reed

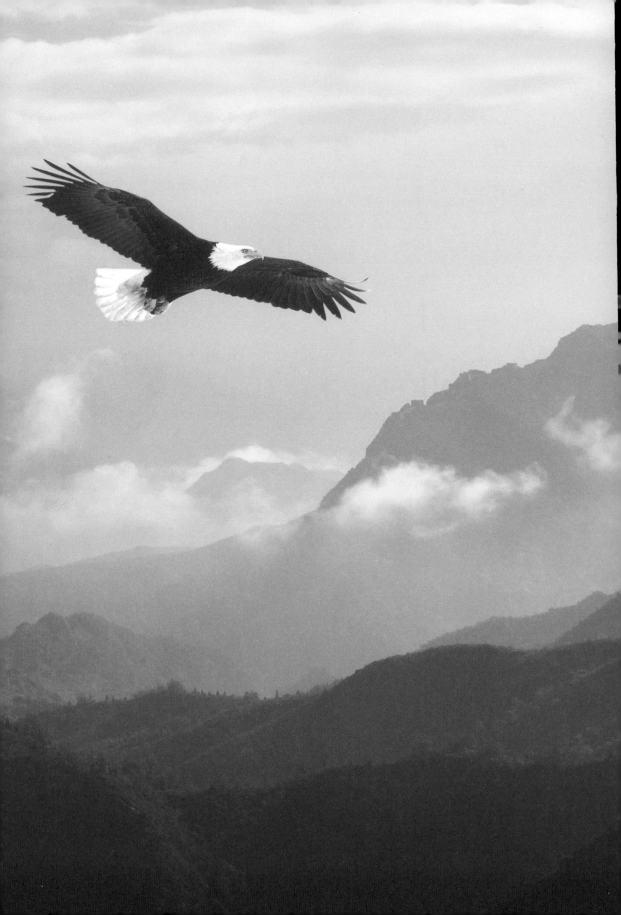

MONTH 12

Follow your dreams

'Remember to celebrate milestones as you prepare for the road ahead'

– Nelson Mandela

In writing this journal you have acknowledged that you have the power to embrace your destiny and shape your future. You know what is best for your body, mind and spirit. No one can live your life, and it is vital that you do what is right for you, not what is right for everyone else.

When I began my wellness journey I wasn't sure where the destination was – I just knew I wanted to make changes and I was willing to put in the time and effort required to live my life more in line with my wellness goals. I took control and faced many fears and made some big life changes that brought me closer each and every day to my desired outcome.

> Nothing changes unless you do, so face your fear of change, embrace the strange, uncomfortable feeling of uncertainty and take action.

My main goal was to do with my health and wellness and I took considerable actions to facilitate change. I started a new form of study, I changed my diet completely, I changed my lifestyle, I changed my expectations and in many ways I dared to dream that I could live a pain-free life.

This month make it your intention to **be in charge of your dreams**. I don't mean the dreams we have at night that we discussed in month ten: I mean your aspirations and hopes. Dreams are bigger than the goals we talked about at the start of this journal. Goals are stepping stones, things that are realistically achievable. Dreams can be bigger than this and at this stage of your year you have proved that you are capable of incredible change.

There are now no limitations on what you can achieve – you can do anything you put your mind to, so why not believe something wonderful will happen today and trust you can make anything happen with your actions. Look within yourself and believe in your own ability to achieve greatness. Don't worry about what is happening in other people's lives – start to live life today as if everything is going your way.

Taking control of your thoughts and actions

Take a moment now to focus on a really big dream. Feel how you would feel if that dream was granted; suspend disbelief and play along, using your imagination. I want you to use the power of intention now to affirm the following statements.

I am in charge of how I feel – today I am going to feel:

1.

2.

3.

4.

5.

I am in charge of my life – it is my dream and ambition to achieve:

1.

2.

3.

4.

5.

'Don't wait for the world to change for you, change it yourself!'

– Kimonui Holgen

Once you have opened yourself up to change and are going in the direction of your dreams, believe in yourself and truly believe you are capable of greatness.

Dream visualisation

Get creative with dream visualisation – this is a mental technique that uses the powers of the **mind** and the **imagination** to manifest what you want.

In simple terms, it is similar to daydreaming: we create imaginary, mental scenarios of events and situations that we want to become factual in the future.

This technique of visualisation for success is used a lot in sports psychology, where performance relates to your mental state as much as your physical state. A sprinter imagines the perfect start and how it will influence their performance; a golfer may picture the perfect swing, over and over again. This form of mental training is often as important as physical practise.

Use your imagination to stay focused on your dreams. Everything starts with your mind, but, as we've said before, you need to conceive it before you can achieve it. Try these tips and tricks to enhance your ability to tap into the power of visualisation.

1. Create a **visualisation board** for your biggest dreams. As you've done previously, show your subconscious images of your goals and your end destination. You have used this technique before so you know what a powerful exercise it is. Look at the board daily, as this will help you attract exactly what you want into your life.
2. **Practise** makes perfect: you need to be consistent and committed to your positive visualisation daily. I recommend just before you go to sleep or early in the morning when your subconscious mind is in control.
3. Be sure to visualise in detail exactly what you want, this will program your subconscious mind and it will begin to attract situations and opportunities to bring your desired outcome into your life more quickly. Don't let fear into the situation by worrying about how it will all fall into place – just for the few minutes that you are using your creative visualisation, **suspend disbelief**.

4. Remember how we used all our senses to live in the moment? Use them again to **focus** on your dreams; experience the feeling of achieving your dream vividly, using all your senses. As well as visualising your dream, you need to **feel** the range of wonderful emotions you will experience when your goal is achieved. Allow your body to truly experience the powerful feelings associated with this experience – imagine what you will hear, see, smell, touch, feel and even say; feel as much as you can to increase the intensity of the emotions. You can do this by remembering how you felt in the past when you achieved something wonderful and bring those feelings into visualising your success and allow yourself to smile with pride and joy as you use your imagination to see your goal manifesting – live in that moment and experience the sheer bliss of the dream.

5. Stay focused and **don't give up**. If you are finding it hard to stay in the moment you can write about what you want and describe the feelings you hope to experience in your journal. Read it before you go to sleep or begin another powerful visualisation. Remember, everything evolves from our thoughts, so believe that you can change energy patterns to bring your goals and desires to you more quickly simply by using your imagination.

WHAT DO YOU WANT?

'Don't wait. The time will never be just right'

– Napoleon Hill

DARE OF THE DAY

Act today as if your dream has already manifested. Live for this day as if you have accomplished your goal

DARE OF THE WEEK

Give yourself the gift of these four words: **I believe in you**.
As the old saying goes, 'If you believe you can or if you believe you can't – **you will**.' So make a conscious effort to believe in yourself this week and write a list of all the things you **believe** you can achieve.

I BELIEVE I CAN ACHIEVE

DARE OF THE MONTH

If you are enjoying the hypnosis relaxations associated with this journal, why not try a little **self-hypnosis** for two to three minutes each day to get you into the right mindset for visualisation. Here is a simple method to follow that you can do anywhere. It is adapted from Emile Coué's method. Coué (1857–1926) was a French psychologist and pharmacist who pioneered self-hypnosis and formulated the laws of suggestion.

Sit in a comfortable chair with your back supported, lie on your bed or a couch, or find anywhere you can relax for a few minutes without being interrupted – somewhere you are comfortable and safe.

Focus your attention on a spot opposite you, slightly above eye level.

Take three deep breaths – slowly. As you inhale your third breath, hold it for the mental count of four full seconds. When you exhale, close your eyes.

As you count backwards ... 4 ... 3 ... 2 ... 1 ... exhale, **relax** and allow yourself to go into a deep, sound, hypnotic rest.

You are to remain in hypnosis for approximately two–three minutes by counting down slowly from twenty-five (25) to one (1). I want you to use your imagination to allow yourself to visualise or imagine each number written on a blackboard and as you count backwards imagine rubbing the number away – see a mental picture of the numbers and see yourself carefully rubbing off the number as you count backwards. In between each count you can repeat your goal silently in your head. Then you simply imagine drawing the next number and repeat rubbing it off and then say your goal again.

I found my mind wandered a lot at the beginning and if it did I started back at the top – at number twenty-five again.

To awaken, when you have reached the number one, take three deep breaths again, hold the last one for the mental count of four and then just count forward from one to four – I mentally say to myself that I am going to awaken refreshed and alert, ready to go about my business in an energetic way.

> **Tip:** To find out more about self hypnosis, you can look up the Émile Coué method

'Happiness is not something ready made; it comes from your own actions'

– Dalai Lama

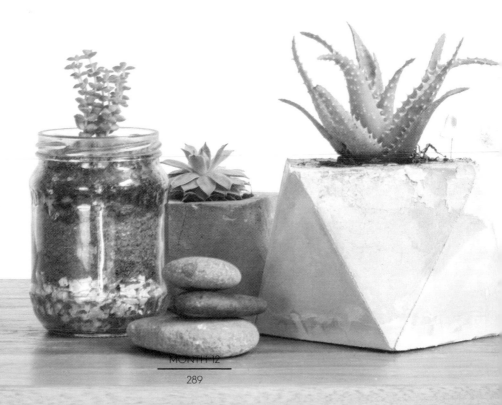

ACHIEVING ONE OF MY GOALS:
extract from my journal

'Look into my eyes, look into my eyes, the eyes, the eyes, not around the eyes, look into my eyes, you're under.'

I am smiling widely as I write this journal entry because I am now a certified hypnotherapist!

*I actually can't believe it and I am **so** proud of myself, although it was a tough few days as I had so much to study and learn for the exams – but they are over and we already know that we have passed! **I am a certified hypnotherapist.** That is something I would never have imagined or dreamed a year ago. I actually cannot believe it. I am not even sure how it all happened, wow. I have to let it all sink in.*

I am not sure what I am going to do with my new qualification but I know it will be something great and exciting. It has helped me so much already, just practising hypnosis and writing my own personalised scripts for pain and wellness.

*I am also currently on **no medication**. I am so **proud** of myself. While people can't see the massive changes on the outside, I still look the same – and in fact it might appear I am doing less work and maybe that I am not as productive as before – but actually I have had a massive transformation. Such a seismic shift in every area of my life, I truly believe that anything is possible now.*

I know one thing for sure – perfecting the art of self-hypnosis on the course has been truly life changing. I have used it consistently for the last three weeks and I have really managed to make great progress. I visualised passing my exams and doing a really great practical exam and today was the fruit of my labour.

I had to use all I have learned today in hypnotising a complete stranger and it was amazing – I had imagined being very calm and in control and that's exactly how I felt today and it really helped me. Just before the practical began I mixed up all my hypnosis scripts – there were so many pages which I hadn't numbered, and I was in a flap trying to gather them all together in preparation. But I just took a deep breath and said my affirmation – 'All is well, everything will turn out perfectly for my higher good and I am safe.'

*I took three minutes to do my self-hypnosis and imagined everything working out perfect and **trusted** I had all the knowledge I needed to pass the exam and complete a perfect practical and calmly carried on with the task at hand.*

It was perfect.

Visualising success, trusting, remaining calm and being brave really carried me through today. I am feeling a little invincible. It is an amazing feeling to know when I began this wellness journey almost a year ago I had no idea I would end up where I am today, but I stuck to the schedule and followed my own instincts and challenged myself and dared to dream I could take control of my life and live the life I wanted to live and today I am now reaping the rewards. I have achieved so much and learned so much along the way and the best thing is I am more eager to learn and I know great possibilities are waiting to be manifested!

So what do I want to manifest next? That's the question I am pondering now.

For tonight I am just so grateful that I passed my exams and I am so thankful I had a great teacher and wonderful friends on the course that inspired and encouraged me along the way. Life is great, when you dare to dream!

'You can't connect the dots looking forward; you can only connect them looking backwards. So you have to trust that the dots will somehow connect in your future. You have to trust in something – your gut, destiny, life, karma, whatever. This approach has never let me down, and it has made all the difference in my life'

– Steve Jobs

MONTHLY REVIEW

This month's hypnosis relaxation will encourage you to dream **big** and follow your heart's true desire.

▸ Some of the most influential people in history kept a journal of their life. Ralph Waldo Emerson wrote a journal about his philosophies, the diaries of Andy Warhol document the artist's day-to-day life, Jane Austen wrote down her ideas for characters and novels and Oprah Winfrey was quoted as saying, 'Keeping a journal will absolutely change your life in ways you've never imagined.'

▸ This is your story – you have the power to write the ending and make it your intention to keep this journal.

▸ If you need to go over any of the lessons learned a great way to reconnect is with the daily hypnosis relaxations which are always on the website and new ones are added all the time.

▸ Be honest about your own feelings in the journal pages and remember the wise words of Socrates 'An unexamined life is not worth living.'

PROMPTS

Make a list of the people in your life that support you and share your dreams:

I really wish others knew this about me:

Name what is enough for you and what you have learned about yourself:

What have I learned from my journal writing?

My Journal

'I never travel without my
diary. One should always have
something sensational to read on
the train.'

— Oscar Wilde

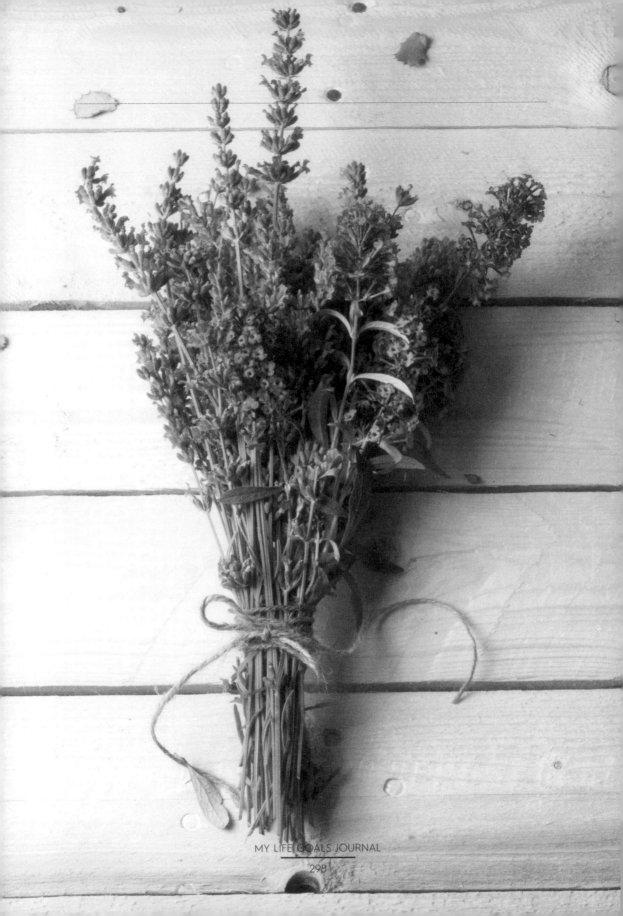

YOUR LIFE
GOALS JOURNAL

The new you

As you near the end of your life goals journal, now is the time to review where you are and reset yourself so you can refocus on the future. The end of the journal is not the end of the journey or of your story: it is just the start. It has prepared you for the next step.

Review

Take time to look back over your journal journey and review how you have achieved great change in each area of your life. Take time to read over your writing – this can be both cathartic and informative. It is illuminating watching the progression of the seeds that you sowed at the beginning take root and bloom. Take time to review each stage.

1. Being the true you and goal setting

_____

_____

_____

2. Love and self-care

_____

_____

_____

3. Thoughts create your reality

_____

_____

_____

4. Conscious eating and healthy living

....

....

....

5. Self-talk

....

....

....

6. Manifestation and abundance

....

....

....

7. Mindfulness and nature

....

....

....

8. Appreciation of life

....

....

....

9. Stress-free living

....

....

....

....

10. Stillness and sleep

....

....

....

....

11. Surrender and let go

....

....

....

....

12. Follow your dreams

....

....

....

....

Reset

Look to the future and apply what you have learned to the months ahead. Create a road map for the year to come.

Decide what you want to achieve in the next twelve months. Instead of wishing and hoping that your goals will come true, you now have the tools to ensure that they will – all you need to do is begin the planning process to see your goals become a reality.

You have harnessed the art of narrowing your focus in the recent months and you have the tools to take your vision of those long-term goals and turn them into achievable, believable and desirable dreams – **you can do it**!

You have all the wisdom and skills required to apply your own inner knowledge so follow your instinct and manifest everything you want. Think positively and allow time for yourself.

If you believe your tomorrow is secure it will make your today so much more enjoyable.

Trust in tomorrow and live in today.

You have taken time to discover your long-term goals and you know you can improve your well-being and overall wellness by following the guidelines outlined here. We can't predict how life will unfold, but you can set goals that provide a sense of meaning, purpose and direction to your life – this is overwhelmingly positive and I hope this journal has allowed you to look forward with optimism and experience every day with more joy.

CREATE A MENTAL MEMORY BOX

Savour the precious moments that make life worth living. Make a list of them here:

Positive psychology pioneer Martin Seligman has identified five elements essential to human well-being using the acronym PERMA.

P is for **positive emotions** such as love, joy, gratitude, awe and inspiration.

E is for **engagement** in activities that are totally absorbing and use your signature strengths.

R is for **relationships** – being authentically connected to others.

M is for **meaning** – living a meaningful life and serving or belonging to something bigger than you.

A is for **accomplishment** – the pursuit of achievement as well as mastery for its own sake.

BUILDING FOR LIFE

Using the PERMA model, create the building blocks for the life you want to live. These will be the foundations of your continued wellness and success. Focus on projects or goals that truly **inspire** you and will uplift your spirit and mind.

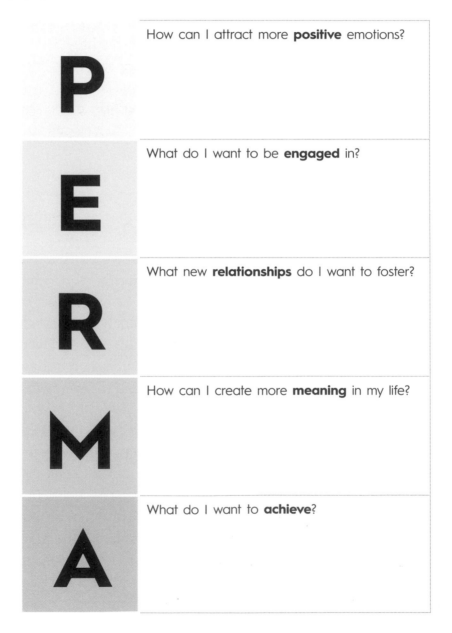

P — How can I attract more **positive** emotions?

E — What do I want to be **engaged** in?

R — What new **relationships** do I want to foster?

M — How can I create more **meaning** in my life?

A — What do I want to **achieve**?

A REMINDER FOR SETTING NEW GOALS FOR THE YEAR AHEAD

Use only **SMART** – specific, measurable, achievable, realistic and timed – goals with **PLAN** – positive feeling, love yourself, attach an action and no excuses!

When you are figuring out your goals, make sure they pass the **PERMA** test so that your well-being will increase.

Remember to be **thankful** for all the blessings in your life.

Visualise clearly what you want to achieve and make sure your thoughts, words and affirmations are positive and focused on your goals.

Believe in yourself and never give up on your own brilliance. Recognise what is great about your life right now trust and believe more joy and success will manifest in your future.

Remember we are all on a journey, so expect some bumps in the road and lots of twists and turns, and have fun and enjoy. It's not about reaching the destination but enjoying the path along the way. Sometimes it's the **journey** that teaches you about your final **destination.**

Keep **journaling** – remember, you can do it your own way: buy a beautiful notebook and continue to record your thoughts and feelings in a special place. Include pictures, draw shapes or images – this is your sacred space to be your authentic self so express your inner being and allow your essence to shine.

Keep journaling to **find the answers** to any questions or concerns you have about your wellness journey and then take a deep breath and listen for a response from your higher self.

My life goals journal became the antidote to all my insecurities and fears; I kept writing until the remedy to any problem or challenge became clear – it has brought me peace of mind and great riches.

I love reading back through my journals. My writing has helped me reflect on where I used to be and where I am now in my life and I know if you keep writing you will find wisdom in your words and direction in your life. You will begin to see your life through new eyes: through the eyes of your true self.

Good luck.

'Fill your paper with the breathings of your heart'

– William Wordsworth

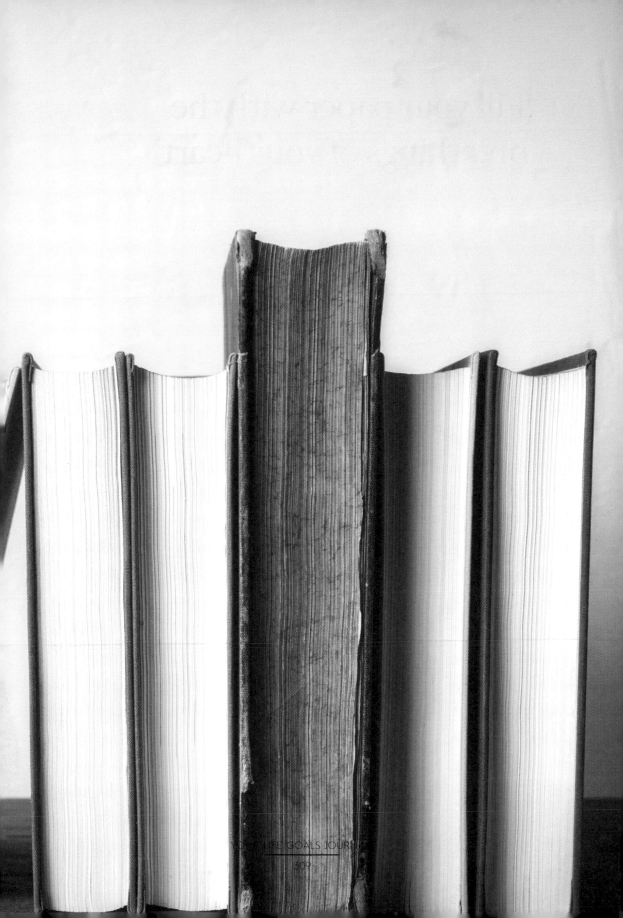

My Journal

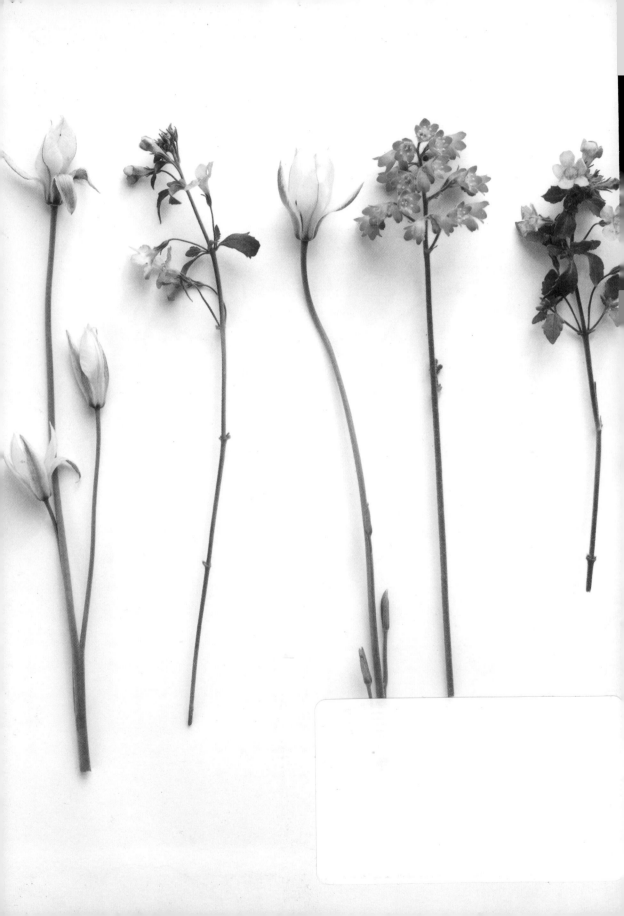